Fetal Monitoring and Assessment

D0357546

Contributors

KAREN J. CRAWLEY, RN, MSN

Department Administrator/Labor and Delivery
Clinical Nurse Specialist
Kaiser Permanente Medical Center
Panorama City, California

EVELYN M. HOM, RN, MS

Perinatal Clinical Nurse Specialist
Perinatal Education Department
Alta Bates Medical Center
Berkeley, California

BRIDGET G. MORAN, RN, MSN

Perinatal Outreach Education Coordinator
Clinical Specialist
Alta Bates Medical Center
Berkeley, California

BARBARA J. PETREE, RN, MA

Private Perinatal Consultant and Educator
Staff Nurse/Labor and Delivery, Antepartum,
High Risk, Postpartum
Stanford University Medical Center
Palo Alto, California

YOLANDA RABELLO, RN, CCRN, MSEd

Coordinator, Antepartum Testing and Perinatal Research
Los Angeles County–University of Southern California
Medical Center
Los Angeles, California

CATHERINE ROMMAL, RNC, BS

Risk Management Education Specialist
Farmers Insurance Group of Companies
Healthcare Professional Liability Division
Malibu, California

Consultants

JANAN BROOMAND, RN, MSN
Staff Nurse II/Labor and Delivery
Kaiser Permanente Medical Center
Walnut Creek, California

JEFF MAIER, MD, FACOG
Perinatologist
The Permanente Medical Group
Walnut Creek, California

JANICE McFADDEN, RN, BSN
Assistant Nurse Manager
Kaiser Permanente Medical Center
Walnut Creek, California

GERALD SAUNDERS, MSc
Health Sciences Librarian
Alta Bates Medical Center
Berkeley, California

Preface

Electronic fetal heart rate monitoring has been in use for over 20 years, and for some reason it seems like yesterday. It continues to be the most commonly used modality for the evaluation of fetal status during the intrapartum and antepartum periods.

The third edition of *Pocket Guide to Fetal Monitoring and Assessment* has been markedly revised in order to provide clinicians with state-of-the-art practical information for use in the clinical setting as well as the basic information for those who are new to electronic fetal heart rate monitoring. The content follows a logical and progressive format in the sequencing of information and is designed for the clinician with a theoretical background in obstetrics. The first chapter provides an overview of perinatal mortality and morbidity and a historical perspective of the art and science of fetal monitoring. The physiological basis for monitoring is explored in Chapter 2. Instrumentation for monitoring is described in Chapter 3 and includes a section on troubleshooting the equipment, as well as considerations to be made before purchasing monitoring equipment. Uterine activity monitoring is described in Chapter 4 and is related to the use of uterine stimulants and tocolytics. Chapters 5 and 6 cover baseline fetal heart rate patterns, periodic changes, unusual patterns, and fetal cardiac dysrhythmias. Reassuring fetal heart rate patterns are contrasted with nonreassuring patterns in Chapter 7; interventions are also presented, including a procedure for amnioinfusion. Chapter 8 covers biophysical and biochemical monitoring techniques, including ultrasound, amniotic fluid index, amniocentesis, procedures on vibroacoustic and nipple-stimulated stress testing, and the application of the biophysical profile. Care of the monitored patient is described in Chapter 9 with a list of factors that should be included in documentation and a checklist for appropriate utilization of the equipment and for interpreting the fetal heart rate pattern. Professional issues discussed in Chapter 10 have been broadened to include discussion of actual litigation, risk management issues, and a chain-of-command for the resolution of conflicts. Appendix A describes the procedure for performing Leopold's maneuvers. Appendix B provides protocols for cervical ripening techniques, amniotomy, and a procedure for the induction and augmentation of labor with oxytocin. Protocols and procedure for the management of preterm labor are provided in Appendix C and cover the use of nifedipine, terbutaline, and other tocolytic agents. Guidelines for care of the patient in labor are provided in Appendix D and use a problem-oriented approach. Appendix E contains selected fetal heart rate patterns for interpretation, demonstrating a methodical approach to evaluating various patterns. Appendix F is a position statement on nursing responsibilities in implementing intrapartum fetal heart rate monitoring, and Appendix G reviews *Nursing Practice Competencies and Educational Guidelines: Antepartum Fetal Surveillance and Intrapartum Fetal Heart Monitoring.* Both are from the Association of Women's Health, Obstetric, and Neonatal Nursing.

The content of this pocket guide provides a single source of information for the care and management of the patient in the labor and delivery suite, the fetal intensive care unit, the LDR/P, and the antepartum inpatient unit or ambulatory care setting where electronic monitoring is employed for fetal surveillance. This book can be and has been used by medical and nursing students, residents, nurse midwives, and registered nurses in the intrapartum and antepartum settings. Input from the users is always welcome by the author to ensure the utility of this book in meeting their needs.

The author wishes to acknowledge the roles of Karrie Tucker Stewart and Jill Tucker in making this book a fruitful and worthwhile endeavor, as they were the impetus for its creation. This book is offered in the hope that those who use it will be instrumental in enhancing the quality of life of the unborn and in promoting the quality of life of the newborn.

Susan Martin Tucker

Contents

Fetal Monitoring and Assessment

Overview of Fetal Monitoring

1

The Problem

The final infant mortality (death before age 1 year) rate for the United States for 1992—8.5 infant deaths per 1000 live-born infants—was the lowest rate ever recorded and represented a decrease of 4.5% from the rate of 8.9 for 1991. This trend in declining infant mortality continues through 1993 with a rate of 8.3. Although we are in the most technically advanced period in perinatology, the fact is that the United States has fallen from twentieth place to twenty-fourth place in infant mortality from 1980 to 1990 (the most recent year for which comparative data are available) among countries or geographic areas with a population of at least 1 million. Some of our largest urban centers continue to have infant mortality rates comparable to those of developing nations. Since 1992 there has been a decrease in deaths from respiratory distress syndrome, adverse effects of accidents, and sudden infant death syndrome. The leading cause of death in white infants was congenital anomalies (about 25%) and for black infants the leading cause of death was disorders related to short gestation and unspecified low birth weight (nearly 18%) (JAMA, 1995). A *Healthy People 2000* national health objective is to reduce the overall infant mortality rate to no more than seven per 1000 live-born infants, which can be achieved by sustaining an average annual decrease of at least 2.4% for the total population.

Strategies to achieve this objective need to consider the various factors accounting for infant mortality in the United States. Improved access to adequate prenatal care and understanding of etiologic risk factors for preterm delivery can contribute to a reduction in mortality from disorders related to short gestation and unspecified low birth weight (LBW). Reducing deaths related to maternal complications of pregnancy will require assessment of the adequacy of

1

the content of care in addition to expanding access to prenatal care. The answer to improving our infant mortality rates is to provide universal access to early maternity and pediatric care for all mothers and infants and in making the health and well-being of mothers and infants a national priority.

This information helps put into perspective the scope of the problem related to neonatal outcomes: that although they may be improved with the use of high-tech equipment during the perinatal and neonatal period, perfect outcomes cannot be guaranteed. Much of the present technology is taken for granted. There is now an array of biophysical, biochemical, and electronic techniques that monitor the fetus through the antepartum and intrapartum periods. It is easy to forget just how recent the developments have been to overcome the relative inaccessibility of the fetus to monitoring and evaluation.

Historical Overview

Fetal heart tones were first heard and described in the seventeenth century. During the next 200 years physicians described fetal heart tones or sounds and uterine souffle in medical journals. Then in 1917 Dr. David Hillis, an obstetrician at the Chicago Lying-In Hospital, reported on the use of a head stethoscope, or fetoscope. The chief of staff at the same institution, Dr. JB DeLee, published a report regarding the use of a similar instrument to auscultate the fetal heart. Controversy developed when Dr. DeLee claimed to have had the idea before Dr. Hillis. The instrument that we know today as the fetoscope became known as the DeLee-Hillis stethoscope and has remained essentially unchanged in design and use.

The move to a higher level of technology was made in 1958 when Dr. Edward Hon of the Yale University School of Medicine published a report on continuous fetal electrocardiographic monitoring from the maternal abdomen. Dr. Caldeyro-Barcia of Uruguay and Dr. Hammacher of Germany reported their observations of fetal heart rate patterns associated with fetal distress in 1966 and 1967, respectively. In 1968 Dr. Ralph Benson et al reported results of the collaborative study commissioned by the National Institute of Neurologic Diseases and Blindness. Some 24,863 deliveries were evaluated, and it was demonstrated that there was no correlation between the fetal heart rate as determined using a fetoscope and neonatal condition, except in the most extreme circumstance. This was almost always fetal bradycardia auscultated before a terminal event. Ten years before Benson, Hon discovered the unreliability of counting fetal heart rate when he asked 15 obstetricians to count several rates from a tape recording of the fetal heart, and found a wide divergence in their counting.

As investigators throughout the world made similar observations of fetal heart rate decelerations and fluctuations from the baseline, a confusing array of terminology developed. At an international conference on fetal heart rate monitoring in December 1971 in New Jersey, and later in March 1972 in Amsterdam, Doctors Hon, Caldeyro-Barcia, and their colleagues developed standard nomenclature for fetal heart rate monitoring. However, agreement on paper speed and universal scales was not reached and remained somewhat variable during the 1970s.

Since the first generation of commercially available fetal monitors in the late 1960s, technological advances have improved the quality and accuracy of the tracing. There is currently a proliferation of electronic fetal heart rate monitors on the market with some variations in capabilities; however, the basic components are the same.

There was widespread acceptance of electronic fetal heart rate monitoring in the 1970s with the majority of patients monitored during all or part of their labors. The hope for this technology was that it could prevent all or most cases of cerebral palsy. In addition, it has been hoped that electronic fetal monitoring would be more sensitive and accurate than intermittent auscultation in detecting fetal heart rate patterns that indicate fetal compromise.

Findings and Controversies

Several studies have indicated that there is either no change or perhaps a slight increase in the incidence of cerebral palsy in the past several years, during which time electronic fetal heart rate monitoring has been in use. It is difficult to determine if improved intrapartum care and appropriate intervention for abnormal heart rate patterns have contributed to a decrease in cerebral palsy, since increased survival rates for very low birth weight infants and improved neonatal care for asphyxiated infants have kept these numbers fairly constant.

Retrospective studies have correlated abnormal fetal heart rate patterns with low Apgar scores, fetal and neonatal acidosis, morbidity, and mortality. The infant mortality rate declined between 1970 and 1987 from 20.0 to 10.1 per 1000 live births. However, during this period the rate of cesarean sections increased because of a variety of factors, including changes in medical practice such as the performance of cesarean sections for breech presentations and the discontinuance of midforceps deliveries. It was suggested that there was a relationship between the increased cesarean section rate and the use of electronic fetal monitors. Governmental and consumer groups were critical of this increase despite the fact that there was an associated decrease in perinatal mortality. Cesarean section rates and VBAC (vaginal birth after cesarean) rates do vary among facilities because of demographic differences and practices at the institution. Another variable is the ability of the staff to interpret patterns. Criticism by groups must be well taken in those facilities where personnel are not well trained and where there are no quality improvement activities such as a review of records by a multidisciplinary team of physicians and nurses for patients undergoing cesarean section for fetal distress based on the interpretation of the fetal monitor pattern.

A recent study has been done to determine whether continuous intrapartum electronic monitoring was associated with decreased perinatal mortality and morbidity compared with intermittent auscultation. A total of 1428 patients were included, with 746 in the electronic fetal monitoring (EFM) group and 682 in the auscultation group. There were no differences between the groups in terms of maternal factors; however, more of the patients monitored electronically received oxytocin for either augmentation or induction. There was a higher incidence of nonreassuring fetal heart rate patterns in the EFM group and a higher rate of surgical intervention. There were no differences in 1- and 5-minute Apgar scores, fetal acidosis, and neonatal factors such as the need for resuscitation, intensive care, use of assisted ventilation, and other complications. There were two neonatal deaths in the EFM group and nine perinatal deaths in the auscultation group (two intrapartum and seven neonatal deaths). The perinatal death rate related to fetal hypoxia was significantly less in the EFM group (0 of 746) versus 6 of 682 in the auscultation group. The conclusion of this controlled trial was that intrapartum EFM as the primary and only method of intrapartum fetal surveillance was associated with decreased perinatal mortality caused by fetal hypoxia but it was also associated with higher rates of surgical intervention for suspected fetal distress (Vintzileos et al, 1993).

The presumption that electronic fetal monitoring would be more sensitive and accurate than intermittent auscultation in detecting fetal heart rate patterns that indicate fetal compromise has been supported by this random prospective study. Yet there are data that support the conclusion that intermittent auscultation is equivalent to continuous electronic fetal monitoring. It must be noted, however, that in the majority of the studies done there was a 1:1 nurse/patient ratio. Because of the fluctuations in the numbers of patients in labor at any one time, it is very difficult, if not impossible, in some settings to provide this type of care from both a staffing and a cost factor standpoint.

Because of the wide acceptance and use of electronic fetal heart rate monitoring in today's busy obstetrical suites, it is doubtful that it will be abandoned in favor of auscultation, primarily because of the associated economic implications related to staffing. Auscultation, however, is a viable alternative to electronic monitoring and will be discussed in Chapter 3.

Physiological Basis for Monitoring

Electronic fetal monitoring (EFM) provides a technique for assessment of uterofetoplacental physiology and the adequacy of fetal oxygenation. Characteristic fetal heart rate (FHR) patterns are demonstrated as the result of hypoxic and nonhypoxic stresses or stimulation to the uterofetoplacental unit. Therefore it is important to have a basic understanding of the factors involved in fetal oxygenation, including uteroplacental circulation and physiology of FHR regulation.

Placenta and Intervillous Space

The placenta serves as a liaison between the fetal and maternal circulations (Figure 2-1). Oxygenated blood is delivered to the fetus through the umbilical vein. Deoxygenated blood returns to the placental chorionic villi through the two umbilical arteries. The chorionic villi are tiny vascular branches of the placenta that extend into the intervillous space. Maternal blood spurts upward from the uterine spiral arterioles and spreads laterally at random into the intervillous space, completely surrounding and bathing the villi (Figure 2-2). Although maternal and fetal blood are separated by a thin membrane and do not mix, several mechanisms occur whereby substances are exchanged across the placental membrane.

Mechanisms Occurring Within Intervillous Space

The intervillous space then acts as a depot for the exchange of oxygen and nutrients and provides for the elimination of waste products. Together with the chorionic villi it functions as a fetal lung,

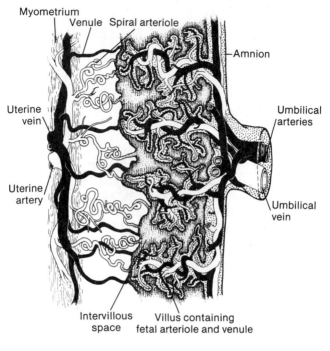

Figure 2-1
Schema of placenta.

gastrointestinal tract, kidney, skin (for heat exchange), infection barrier, and moderator of acid-base balance (Table 2-1).

At term some 700 to 800 ml of blood (10% to 15% of maternal cardiac output) perfuses the uterus each minute. Approximately 80% of this is within the intervillous space.

Exchange of Gases

Transport and transfer of respiratory gases are of critical importance to fetal survival. Oxygen and carbon dioxide exchange are complex processes that depend on many physiological and biochemical factors. These include intervillous space blood flow, diffusing capacity of the placenta, placental area and vascularity, membrane perme-

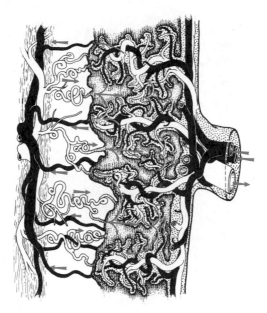

Figure 2-2
As maternal blood enters the intervillous space, it spurts
upward from uterine spiral arterioles and spreads laterally at
random.

ability and thickness, oxygen tension of uterine and umbilical blood
vessels, hemoglobin affinity and hemoglobin concentration of maternal and fetal blood, and fetal umbilical cord blood flow. Intervillous space blood flow has already been described. Further description of the other factors follows.

Diffusing Capacity of Placenta

The diffusing capacity of the placenta regulates the rate of oxygen
transfer by a concentration gradient and the rate of blood flow. Oxygen diffuses from the maternal blood, which has a higher partial
pressure, to the fetal blood, which has a lower partial pressure. Maternal and fetal blood flow rates can be altered by decreases in maternal blood pressure (as occurs with supine hypotension and following conduction anesthesia such as spinal, caudal, or epidural
anesthesia); maternal exercise, uterine hypertonus or polysystole,

Table 2-1   Mechanisms occurring within intervillous space

Mechanism	Description	Substances
Diffusion	Passage of substances from a region of higher concentration to one of lower concentration along a concentration gradient that is passive and requires no energy	Oxygen Carbon dioxide Small ions (sodium, chloride) Lipids Fat-soluble vitamins Many drugs
Facilitated diffusion	Substances pass on the basis of a concentration gradient, probably a carrier molecule	Glucose Carbohydrates
Active transport	Passage of substances from one area to another against a concentration gradient; carrier molecules and energy are required	Amino acids Water-soluble vitamins Large ions (calcium, iron, iodine)
Bulk flow	Transfer of substances by a hydrostatic or osmotic gradient	Water Dissolved electrolytes
Pinocytosis	Transfer of minute, engulfed particles across a cell	Immune globulins Serum proteins
Breaks or leakage	Small defects in the placental membrane allowing for passage of substances	Maternal or fetal blood cells and plasma (potentially resulting in isoimmunization)

decreased placental surface area (abruptio placentae or infarcts); or by increases in blood pressure, such as occurs with preeclampsia or vasoconstricting drugs.

Placental Area

The larger and more vascular the placenta, the greater amount of substances that can be transferred between mother and fetus. Reduced placental area is associated with maternal hypertension, maternal diabetes, maternal vascular disease, fetal growth retardation, intrauterine infection, abruptio placentae, placenta previa, placental infarctions, and circumvallate placenta.

Oxygen Tension

Oxygen tension in maternal arterial blood is determined by adequate pulmonary function. Diminished function resulting from maternal disease process or hypoventilation will decrease arterial oxygen tension (arterial P_{O_2}). This can be remedied by adding inspired oxygen.

Oxygen transfer from maternal to fetal hemoglobin is regulated by the oxygen tension of the umbilical blood vessels. Generally, oxygen tension of the umbilical vessels is much lower than that of the maternal vessels (Figure 2-3). Some factors that compensate for this low fetal oxygen tension follow:

1. Increased fetal cardiac output (three to four times that of the resting adult per kilogram of body weight) based on heart rate
2. Increased oxygen-carrying capacity caused by high hemoglobin values (as compared with adult blood)
3. Increased affinity of fetal blood for oxygen (as compared with adult blood) with a higher saturation of fetal hemoglobin at the same given P_{O_2} based on the fetal hemoglobin dissociation curve
4. Anatomical fetal shunts: ductus venosus, foramen ovale, and ductus arteriosis

Hemoglobin and Oxygen Affinity

Hemoglobin concentrations of maternal and fetal blood differ at term. Maternal hemoglobin is approximately 12 g/100 ml, in contrast with fetal hemoglobin, which is about 15 g/100 ml. Each gram of hemoglobin is capable of combining with 1.34 ml of oxygen. This increased oxygen-carrying capacity of fetal blood plus the high affinity of fetal blood for oxygen facilitate the transfer of oxygen from mother to fetus.

Umbilical Blood Flow

The mechanical force of a uterine contraction impedes intervillous space blood flow, exerts pressure directly on the fetus, and can occlude blood flow in both directions through the umbilical cord. Rapid fetal asphyxia with hypoxemia and acidosis can occur with entrapment and compression of the cord between fetal parts and the uterine wall. Transient cord compression occurs in about 40% of all labors, and the fetus is usually able to compensate in the intervals between contractions. However, in some labors in which the cord

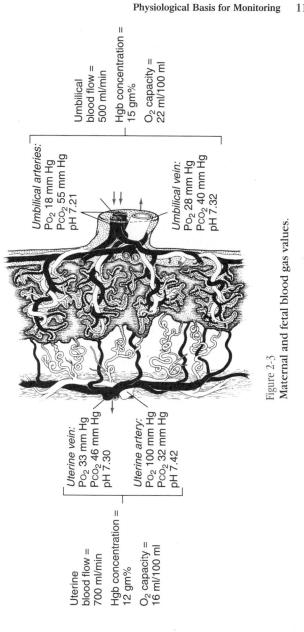

Umbilical
blood flow =
500 ml/min

Hgb concentration =
15 gm%

O_2 capacity =
22 ml/100 ml

Umbilical arteries:
Po_2 18 mm Hg
Pco_2 55 mm Hg
pH 7.21

Umbilical vein:
Po_2 28 mm Hg
Pco_2 40 mm Hg
pH 7.32

Uterine vein:
Po_2 33 mm Hg
Pco_2 46 mm Hg
pH 7.30

Uterine artery:
Po_2 100 mm Hg
Pco_2 32 mm Hg
pH 7.42

Uterine
blood flow =
700 ml/min

Hgb concentration =
12 gm%

O_2 capacity =
16 ml/100 ml

Figure 2-3
Maternal and fetal blood gas values.

prolapses or is short, knotted, wrapped around fetal body parts, or where oligohydramnios is present, uncorrectable and prolonged variable deceleration of the fetal heart rate occurs. This is an obstetrical emergency, usually requiring immediate operative intervention, since fetal asphyxiation and death can occur. Amnioinfusion, the instillation of normal saline through an intrauterine catheter (a discussion of which can be found in Chapter 7), can act as a buffer between fetal parts and the uterine wall and can relieve variable decelerations caused by cord compression.

Decreased Uterine Blood Flow

Uterine blood flow is determined by uterine arterial and venous pressure and uterine vascular resistance. Some causes of decreased uterine blood flow follow.

Maternal Position

A decrease in blood flow to the uterus can occur when the mother is in the dorsal recumbent position. The gravid uterus lies on the mother's vertebral column, exerting pressure on the great vessels, particularly the inferior vena cava. This pressure can compress the vessel, decreasing the volume of blood returning to the heart and producing a decrease in maternal cardiac output, hypotension, and a decrease in uterine blood flow. This mechanism is called *supine hypotension syndrome.*

Exercise

Fetal tachycardia that occurs after maternal exercise is thought to be caused by a transitory period of reduced fetal oxygenation. Although maternal exercise diverts blood to the muscle groups and away from the uterus, there is no evidence that exercise is harmful when there is normal uteroplacental function.

Uterine Contractions

Uterine contractions cause a decrease in the rate of perfusion of maternal blood through the intervillous space. Angiographic studies demonstrating this have shown impaired filling of the lobules with contrast medium during uterine contractions. In addition, fetal arterial blood oxygen tension decreases following the onset of each uterine contraction. The fetus, in most gestations, seems well able to compensate for these relatively minor stresses. However, in high-risk pregnancies in which the margin of fetal reserve is abnormally low, uterine contractions can cause some degree of hypoxia and commensurate decreases in the fetal heart rate, known as late decelerations. Recognition and treatment of late decelerations are described in Chapter 6.

To avoid compounding these stresses, it is important that the uterus relax adequately between contractions, that contractions not be excessively long, and that the tonus not rise. Intrauterine pressure between contractions—*resting tone (tonus)*—ranges from 5 to 15 mm Hg, with the average pressure between 8 and 12 mm Hg. During contractions intrauterine pressure ranges from 30 to more than 80 mm Hg, with an intensity of 50 to more than 100 mm Hg at the peak of the contraction. Angiographic studies show a cessation of maternal blood flow to the intervillous space with intrauterine pressures of 50 to 60 mm Hg during normal labor contractions.

It is thought that the fetus receives most of the oxygen and nutrients and eliminates most of the carbon dioxide (CO_2) between contractions while the uterus is at rest. Thus a healthy fetus with a normal placenta subjected to frequent contractions with inadequate uterine relaxation can become hypoxic and acidotic.

Uterine Hypertonus

Uterine hypertonus—excessively high intrauterine pressure—can also cause the fetus to experience stress. Uterine hypertonus may occur spontaneously in some patients, particularly in those with a very distended uterus, as a result of hydramnios, multiple gestation, or macrosomia. However, hypertonus is most frequently caused by uterine hyperstimulation with oxytocin (Schmidt, 1993). In some sensitive patients oxytocin produces hypertonus, characterized by high intrauterine pressure with absence of relaxation for a prolonged period. Abruptio placentae may also cause uterine hypertonus as a result of irritation of the myometrium from extravasated blood. In preeclampsia uterine resting tone is elevated because of vasoconstriction, decreased uterine blood flow, and reduced placental surface area (Freeman, 1991). In addition, the following factors can interfere with placental perfusion and jeopardize the fetus:

1. Contractions lasting longer than 90 seconds
2. Periods of relaxation between contractions that are less than 30 seconds
3. Inadequate decrease in intrauterine pressure between contractions

Surface Area of Placenta

The potential for fetal hypoxia is increased with any reduction in the placental surface area. Abruptio placentae is a clear example of this. Reduced placental area exposes the fetus to uteroplacental insufficiency and is associated with infarcts (as in hypertensive or prolonged pregnancies), maternal vascular disease, maternal diabetes, intrauterine infection, placenta previa, or circumvallate placenta.

Conduction Anesthesia

Maternal hypotension caused by sympathetic blockade occurring with conduction anesthesia reduces blood flow in the intervillous space. Restoration of uterine blood flow is usually achieved by positional changes and expansion of maternal blood volume. Prehydration for women who are about to receive conduction anesthesia should be considered. Pressor agents, such as ephedrine, may also be required to restore maternal blood pressure.

Hypertension

Whether maternal hypertension is essential or pregnancy-induced, there is an increase in vascular resistance, resulting in a decrease in uterine blood flow.

Physiology of Fetal Heart Rate Regulation

The average fetal heart rate at term is 140 beats per minute (bpm). The normal range is 120 to 160 bpm. Earlier in gestation the fetal heart rate is slightly higher, with the average being approximately 160 bpm at 20 weeks' gestation (Freeman, 1991). The rate progressively decreases as the fetus reaches term.

The heart rate is normally modulated by the sympathetic and parasympathetic nervous systems based on baroceptor and chemoceptor response (Figure 2-4). Regulatory control also depends on other factors, as described in Table 2-2.

Other factors that may influence the fetal heart rate are disturbances such as hyperthermia tachycardia and hypothermia bradycardia (Schmidt, 1993).

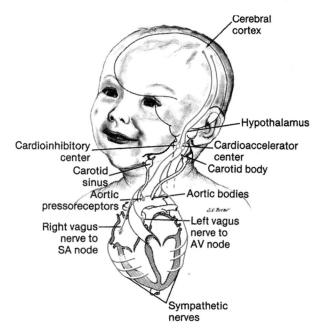

Figure 2-4
Schema of relation of control of FHR from central nervous
system, parasympathetic and sympathetic divisions of
autonomic nervous system, baroceptors, and chemoceptors.

Table 2-2   Regulatory control of fetal heart rate

Factors Regulating Fetal Heart Rate	Location
Parasympathetic division of autonomic nerve system	Vagus nerve fibers supply sinoatrial (SA) and atrioventricular (AV) node
Sympathetic division of autonomic nervous system	Nerves widely distributed in myocardium
Baroceptors	Stretch receptors in aortic arch and carotid sinus at the junction of the internal and external carotid arteries
Chemoceptors	Peripheral—in carotid and aortic bodies

Central—in medulla oblongata |
| Central nervous system | Cerebral cortex

Hypothalamus

Medulla oblongata |
| Hormonal regulation | Adrenal medulla |

Action	Effect
Stimulation causes release of acetylcholine at myoneural synapse	Decreases FHR Maintains beat-to-beat variability
Stimulation causes release of norepinephrine at synapse	Increases FHR Increases strength of myocardial contraction Increases cardiac output
Responds to increase in blood pressure by stimulating stretch receptors to send impulses via vagus or glossopharyngeal nerve to midbrain, producing vagal response and slowing heart activity	Decreases FHR Decreases blood pressure Decreases cardiac output
Responds to a marked peripheral decrease in O_2 and increase in CO_2	Produces bradycardia, sometimes with increased variability
Central chemoceptors respond to decreases in O_2 tension and increases in CO_2 tension in blood and/or cerebrospinal fluid	Produces tachycardia and increase in blood pressure with decrease in variability
Responds to fetal movement	Increases reactivity and variability
Responds to fetal sleep	Decreases reactivity and variability
Regulates and coordinates autonomic activities (sympathetic and parasympathetic)	
Mediates cardiac and vasomotor reflex center by controlling heart action and blood vessel diameter	Maintains balance between cardioacceleration and cardiodeceleration
Releases epinephrine and norepinephrine with severe fetal hypoxia producing sympathetic response	Increases FHR Increases strength of myocardial contraction and blood pressure Increases cardiac output

Continued

Table 2-2   Regulatory control of fetal heart rate—cont'd

Factors Regulating Fetal Heart Rate	Location
Hormonal regulation, cont'd	Adrenal cortex
	Vasopressin (plasma catecholamine)
Blood volume/capillary fluid shift	Fluid shift between capillaries and interstitial spaces
Intraplacental pressures	Intervillous space
Frank-Starling mechanism	Based on stretching of myocardium by increased inflow of venous blood into right atrium

Action	Effect
Low fetal blood pressure stimulates release of aldosterone, decreases sodium output, increases water retention, which increases circulating blood volume	Maintains homeostasis of blood volume
Produces vasoconstriction of nonvital vascular beds in the asphyxiated fetus	Distributes blood flow to maintain FHR and variability
Responds to elevated blood pressure by causing fluid to move out of capillaries and into interstitial spaces	Decreases blood volume and blood pressure
Responds to low blood pressure by causing fluid to move out of interstitial space into capillaries	Increases blood volume and blood pressure
Fluid shift between fetal and maternal blood is based on osmotic and blood pressure gradients; maternal blood pressure is about 100 mm Hg and fetal blood pressure about 55 mm Hg; therefore balance is probably maintained by some compensatory factor	Regulates blood volume and blood pressure
In the adult the myocardium is stretched by an increased inflow of blood, causing the heart to contract with greater force than before and pump out more blood; the adult then is able to increase cardiac output by increasing heart rate and stroke volume; this mechanism is not well-developed in the fetus	Cardiac output is dependent on heart rate in the fetus: $\downarrow$ FHR = $\downarrow$ cardiac output $\uparrow$ FHR = $\uparrow$ cardiac output

Instrumentation for Fetal Heart Rate and Uterine Activity Monitoring

3

Overview

The goal of fetal heart rate monitoring is to detect signs that warn of potential adverse events in order to provide intervention in a timely manner. The fetal heart rate can be monitored by intermittent auscultation or by electronic means with an external or internal device. This chapter presents a description of devices that can be used to monitor the fetal heart rate and includes information on uterine activity monitoring, central display terminals, and telemetry. In addition, factors to be considered before purchasing an electronic monitor are provided.

Auscultation of Fetal Heart Rate

Description

In addition to the use of the electronic fetal monitor, auscultation of the fetal heart rate can be performed with a stethoscope, DeLee-Hillis fetoscope, or Doppler ultrasound device. If a *stethoscope* is used, the end should be turned so that the domed side of the stethoscope, rather than the flat side, is open to the connective tubing to the ear pieces. The domed side is then placed on the maternal abdomen. The *fetoscope* should be applied over the listener's head, since bone conduction amplifies the fetal heart sounds for counting. It is the ventricular fetal heart sounds that can be counted with the stethoscope and fetoscope. The *Doppler ultrasound* device transmits ultra-high frequency sound waves to the moving interface of the fetal heart valves and deflects these back to the device, converting them into an electronic signal that can be counted.

Procedure	Rationale
1. Perform Leopold's maneuvers (see Appendix A) by palpating the maternal abdomen	1. To identify fetal presentation and position
2. Place the listening device over the area of maximum intensity and clarity of the fetal heart sounds, which is usually over the back of the fetus	2. To obtain the clearest and loudest sound, which is easier to count
3. Count the maternal radial pulse	3. To differentiate it from the fetal rate
4. Palpate the abdomen for the absence of uterine activity	4. To be able to count FHR between contractions
5. Count the fetal heart rate (FHR) for 30 to 60 seconds *between* contractions	5. To identify the baseline rate, which can only be assessed during the absence of uterine activity
6. Auscultate the FHR during a contraction and for 30 seconds after the end of the contraction	6. To identify the FHR during the contraction and as a response to the contraction
7. When there are distinct discrepancies in FHR during or between listening periods, auscultate for a longer period, both during, after, and between contractions	7. To identify changes from the baseline that indicate the need for another mode of FHR monitoring

Frequency of Auscultation

Intermittent auscultation of the fetal heart rate should be performed at 15-minute intervals during the first stage of active labor and at 5-minute intervals during the second stage of labor. In well-controlled research studies this frequency has been shown to be equivalent to continuous electronic monitoring in the assessment of the fetal condition in pregnancies with risk factors. These studies did employ a *ratio of one nurse to one patient,* which should be employed if aus-

cultation is used as the primary technique of fetal heart rate surveillance. In low-risk pregnancies the standard practice is to evaluate and record the fetal heart rate at least every 30 minutes in the
active phase of the first stage of labor and at least every 15 minutes
in the second stage. However, because 20% of perinatal morbidity
and mortality arises during the intrapartum period from patients who
have no complications during their pregnancies (ACOG/AAP,
1992), it may be more prudent to auscultate the FHR at more frequent intervals.

   Auscultation of the FHR should occur *before* the administration
of medications (including oxytocics and analgesics) and anesthetics,
before periods of ambulation, and before artificial rupture of membranes. The FHR should be assessed immediately *following* rupture
of membranes, changes in strength of uterine contraction (resting
tone increase, sustained contraction, or tachysystole), vaginal examinations, changes in dosage of oxytocics, response to oxytocics,
administration of medications (during peak action period), urinary
catheterization, periods of ambulation, changes in dosage of anesthetic agents, and response to analgesics and anesthetics.

Documentation

Documentation of the fetal heart rate must be accompanied by other
routine parameters that are assessed during labor, including uterine
activity, maternal observations and assessment, and both maternal
and fetal responses to interventions. It should be noted how long
the heart rate was auscultated and whether this was before, during,
and/or immediately after a uterine contraction. The rate, rhythm,
and abrupt or gradual increases or decreases of the FHR during any
part of this auscultated period should be described in relationship
to the concurrent uterine activity. It is not appropriate to describe
auscultated FHR using the descriptive terms associated with electronic fetal monitoring because the majority of the terms are visual
descriptions of the patterns produced on the monitor tracing (e.g.,
early, late, and variable decelerations). However, terms that are nu-
merically defined, such as bradycardia and tachycardia, can be used.

Interpretation
Reassuring fetal heart rate:

   - FHR in the normal heart rate range without wide fluctuations
     from the average rate (which is obtained between contractions)
     usually over a 10-minute period of time

nreassuring fetal heart rate:

An average FHR between contractions of less than 100 bpm
A FHR drop of 10 to 30 bpm below the baseline 20 to 30 seconds after a contraction
Unexplained FHR of more than 160 bpm (tachycardia), especially if this occurs through three or more contractions in an at-risk patient

Management Options of a Nonreassuring Fetal Heart Rate

- Continuous electronic fetal monitoring (preferably internal) to validate FHR pattern. (This should be strongly considered for conditions that identify the fetus at risk for antepartum and/or intrapartum perinatal hypoxia or asphyxia. See the box below.)
- Fetal scalp sampling for pH

High-Risk Conditions for Fetal Hypoxia/Asphyxia[*]

Postdates pregnancy
Pregnancy-induced hypertension or preeclampsia
Chronic hypertension
Diabetes mellitus
Intrauterine growth retardation
Preterm labor
Preterm rupture of membranes
Chronic renal disease
Active pulmonary disease
Cyanotic heart disease
Third trimester bleeding
Lupus or collagen vascular disease
Maternal anemia
Rh isoimmunization
Multiple gestation
Malpresentation
Hydramnios
Oligohydramnios
Meconium-stained amniotic fluid
Abnormal FHR on auscultation

[*] List is not all inclusive.

- Vibroacoustic stimulation with electronic monitoring to assess fetal response

If nonreassuring patterns persist after attempts to correct them have been made, or if ancillary tests are not available or appropriate, then an expeditious delivery may be considered by the physician.

Advantages of Auscultatory Fetal Heart Rate Monitoring

- Widely available and easy to use
- Noninvasive
- Inexpensive
- The sound of fetal heart rate confirms fetal life

Limitations

- May require maternal supine position, which could predispose to supine hypotension syndrome
- Does not provide a permanent, documented record
- The counting of FHR is intermittent
- Cannot assess FHR variability
- Nonreassuring events may occur during unmonitored periods
- Does not allow for early detection of nonreassuring patterns
- Can miss shallow, late decelerations that are associated with hypoxia

In summary, auscultatory fetal heart rate monitoring has been found to be effective if performed in a consistent manner by a nurse caring for one patient according to the prescribed frequency. Because of the time and (nursing) labor-intensive nature of this method of monitoring, it may not always be an option in a busy unit that has the capability of continuous electronic fetal heart rate monitoring.

Electronic Fetal Monitoring

There are two modes of electronic monitoring. The external, or in-direct, mode employs the use of external transducers placed on the maternal abdominal wall to assess FHR and uterine activity. The internal, or direct, mode uses a spiral electrode to assess the fetal heart rate and variability and the intrauterine catheter to assess uterine activity and intrauterine pressure. A brief description contrasting the external and internal modes of monitoring (Figures 3-1 and 3-2) with a more detailed explanation of application and use follows.

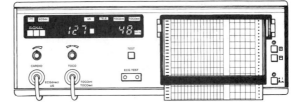

Figure 3-1
Electronic fetal monitor.

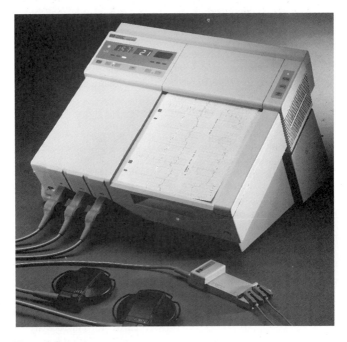

Figure 3-2
The HP 50 IP fetal monitor (Hewlett-Packard) offers internal and external monitoring capabilities including Doppler-detected gross fetal body movements and dual-ultrasound twin monitoring. This model also has a barcode reader that allows routine notations to be entered directly on the tracing.
(Courtesy Hewlett-Packard Company, Böblingen, Germany.)

	External Mode (Indirect)	Internal Mode (Direct)
Fetal heart rate	Ultrasound (Doppler) transducer: High-frequency sound waves reflect mechanical action of fetal heart (easiest and most reliable external method to use during the antepartum and intrapartum periods) Abdominal electrodes: Fetal ECG is obtained when electrodes are properly positioned; it is not currently used for antepartum monitoring because of ease and reliability of ultrasound transducer	Spiral electrode: Electrode converts fetal ECG as obtained from presenting part to FHR via cardiotachometer by measuring consecutive fetal R waves; this method can be used only when membranes are ruptured and the cervix is sufficiently dilated during the intrapartum period; electrode penetrates fetal presenting part 1.5 mm and must be securely attached to ensure a good signal
Uterine activity	Tocotransducer: This instrument monitors frequency and duration of contractions by means of a pressure-sensing device applied to the abdomen; it can be used during antepartum and intrapartum periods	Intrauterine catheter: This instrument monitors frequency, duration, and *intensity* of contractions; the catheter is compressed during contractions, placing pressure on a transducer tip or a strain gauge mechanism of a fluid-filled catheter and then converting the pressure into mm Hg on the uterine activity panel of the strip chart; it can be used only when membranes are ruptured and the cervix is sufficiently dilated during intrapartum period; these catheters are available with a second lumen that can be used for amnioinfusion

External Mode of Monitoring

Ultrasound transducer

Description

Ultrasonic high-frequency sound waves are transmitted by a transducer placed on the maternal abdomen (Figure 3-3). As the ultrasound strikes a moving interface—in this case the fetal heart ventricles—a signal is directed back to the transducer, activating a tachometer. The FHR is printed out on the upper part of the strip chart, and a simultaneous indicator light or audible beep on the monitor is activated with each heartbeat. This Doppler signal can be affected by changes in the position of the transducer or the fetus. Changes in the direction of the sound beam during uterine contractions may distort the tracing and mask periodic changes in the FHR. Because ultrasound reflects mechanical movement of the fetal heart, it cannot assess accurate short-term variability in the FHR. However, monitors with autocorrection capability very closely approximate accurate short-term variability. Some monitors have dual ultrasound channels for the simultaneous monitoring of twins (Figures 3-4 and 3-5).

The ultrasound transducer can be used to monitor FHR during both the antepartum and intrapartum periods. Correct placement of the ultrasound transducer depends on maternal cooperation and operator skill, since the transducer usually needs to be repositioned when the maternal position changes. Excessive fetal movement can

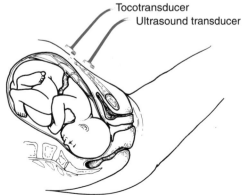

Tocotransducer
Ultrasound transducer

Figure 3-3
Placement of external transducers.

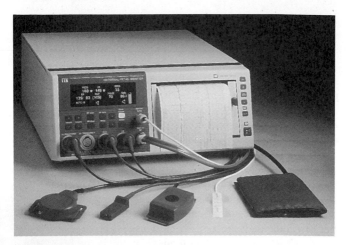

Figure 3-4

Corometrics Model 118 monitor provides internal and external fetal heart rate monitoring as well as maternal pulse oximetry and/or noninvasive blood pressure monitoring.
(Courtesy Corometrics Medical Systems, Inc., Wallingford, Conn.)

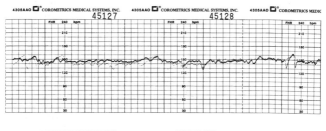

Figure 3-5

Dual ultrasonic heart rate monitoring strip demonstrates the simultaneous external monitoring of twins.
(Courtesy Corometrics Medical Systems, Inc., Wallingford, Conn.)

cause erratic operation of the FHR stylus. Very rapid changes in FHR, such as sudden variable decelerations, may not be followed completely by the ultrasound transducer.

The following information provides a step-by-step approach for use of the ultrasound transducer.

Procedure	Rationale
1. Explain the procedure to the patient and her family	1. To allay anxiety
2. Gather necessary equipment: fetal monitor, ultrasound transducer, and either tocotransducer or intrauterine catheter apparatuses (to assess uterine activity), ultrasonic coupling gel, and abdominal belt	2. To ensure that all equipment is readily accessible
3. Position the patient in a semilateral position of comfort	3. To avoid supine hypotension syndrome
4. Perform Leopold's maneuvers	4. To determine fetal position
5. Insert the ultrasound transducer plug into the appropriate monitor connector labeled "ultrasound" or "cardio"	5. To connect cable plug to appropriate outlet
6. Plug the power cord into the electrical outlet; turn on the power, and gently touch the ultrasound diaphragm to elicit an equal audio response	6. To check for proper functioning of the transducer by simulating fetal heart sounds
7. Apply ultrasound coupling gel to the underside of the transducer placed on the maternal abdomen	7. To aid in the transmission of ultrasound waves (ECG paste frequently occludes this)
8. Place the transducer on the abdomen below the level of the umbilicus in a full-term pregnancy of cephalic presentation or above the level of the umbilicus in a full-term pregnancy of breech presentation	8. To search for the clearest signal, which is obtained by placing the transducer over the location of the fetal heart

Procedure	Rationale
9. Turn the audio-volume control knob while moving the transducer over the abdomen	9. To obtain the strongest fetal signal
10. Secure the ultrasound transducer with the abdominal belt or other fixation device	10. To prevent displacement of transducer
11. Observe the indicator signal, which will flash simultaneously with each fetal heartbeat	11. To verify clarity of input and ensure correct placement of the transducer
12. Set the recorder at 3 cm/min paper speed and observe the FHR on the strip chart; obtain the baseline FHR *between* contractions or periodic changes	12. To ensure that paper feeds correctly and that recording is clear
13. Depress the test button for 10 seconds and make a notation of this on the tracing; ensure that the correct time is printed on the monitor strip (reset monitor clock as necessary) (Figure 3-6)	13. To ensure that the monitor prints out a predetermined number, usually 120 bpm on the corresponding line of the chart paper according to guidelines in manufacturer's operating manual
14. Periodically clean the transducer and maternal abdomen with a damp cloth to remove dried gel; reapply ultrasonic coupling gel and use talcum powder to dust under the abdominal belt if this is the fixation device	14. To keep the skin dry and promote the patient's comfort
15. Reposition the transducer whenever the fetal signal becomes unclear, such as when the mother moves or when the fetus descends in the pelvis	15. To ensure a clear, interpretable tracing during fetal monitoring

Procedure	Rationale
16. When removing the ultra-sound transducer, exercise caution so that it is not dropped or allowed to swing against any equipment; clean the transducer according to the procedure of the facility, or follow the directions in the manufacturer's operating manual (do not use alcohol)	16. To protect the ultrasound crystals from damage
17. Loosely coil the cable and secure with a rubber band or place loosely coiled in a secure area	17. To prevent damage to the wires, which can occur with tight coiling, resulting in loss of or an inadequate fetal signal
18. Dispose of disposable abdominal belt; wash reusable belt according to the facility's procedure before the next patient's use	18. To ensure that disposable belt is not reused and that reusable belt is cleaned and ready for future use

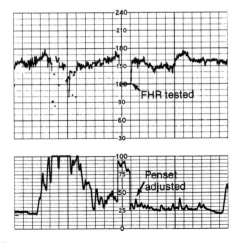

Figure 3-6
Testing of monitor: ultrasound and tocotransducer.

Advantages of the ultrasound transducer

- Noninvasive
- Easy to apply
- May be used during the antepartum period
- Does not require ruptured membranes or cervical dilatation
- No known hazards to mother or fetus
- Provides permanent record of FHR
- Can differentiate FHR from maternal heart rate (eliminating errors due to displacement)

Limitations

- Requires patient cooperation in restricting some movement
- Requires repositioning with fetal or maternal position change that results in loss of signal
- Can assess long-term variability but not short-term variability
- May double-count a slow FHR of less than 60 bpm (because of the inability to distinguish the first from the second heart sound so that they are both counted as equals)*
- May half-count a tachydysrhythmia of more than 180 bpm (because of the inability to reset, which can result in the skipping or elimination of every other heartbeat)*
- Maternal heart rate may be counted if the ultrasound transducer is placed over the maternal arterial vessels, such as the aorta
- Obese patients may be difficult to monitor because of the distance between the transducer and the fetal heart

Abdominal ECG transducer

The abdominal ECG transducer is capable of obtaining the FHR through the maternal abdominal wall. However, it is rarely used due to the time required to obtain an interpretable tracing as a result of fastidious skin preparation and electrode placement. The advantages of the ultrasound transducer far outweigh the utility of the abdominal ECG.

Limitations

- Maternal movement and muscle activity may interfere with the tracing
- Data may be lost when maternal and fetal signals occur at the same moment
- Very difficult to obtain a consistently clear tracing

* Auscultation can verify monitor double/half count.

Tocotransducer (tocodynamometer)
Description

The tocotransducer monitors uterine activity transabdominally by means of a pressure-sensing button that is depressed by uterine contractions or fetal movement. The uterine activity panel of the chart paper displays relative frequency and duration of contractions. Absolute intensity can be assessed only with the intrauterine catheter. The tocotransducer can be used to monitor uterine activity during both the antepartum and intrapartum periods.

A sequential format for use of the tocotransducer is provided below.

Procedure	Rationale
1. Explain the procedure to the patient and her family	1. To allay anxiety
2. Gather the necessary equipment: fetal monitor, tocotransducer (tocodynamometer), and the equipment desired to monitor the FHR	2. To ensure that all equipment is readily accessible
3. Position the abdominal belt around the patient's upper abdomen, over the upper uterine segment, and place her in a semilateral position of comfort	3. To avoid supine hypotension syndrome
4. Insert the tocotransducer plug into the appropriate monitor connector labeled "uterine activity," "toco," or "utero"	4. To connect cable plug to appropriate outlet
5. Place the transducer on the maternal abdomen over the upper uterine segment where there is the least amount of maternal tissue between the pressure-sensing button and the uterus (where uterine contractions are best palpated)	5. To ensure that the upper uterine segment is as close as possible to the pressure-sensing button
6. Secure the tocotransducer with the abdominal belt	6. To prevent displacement of the transducer

Procedure	Rationale
7. Set the recorder at 3 cm/min paper speed, check the printed time/date for accuracy, and observe the strip chart	7. To ensure that the paper feeds correctly and that recording is clear
8. Adjust the sensitivity calibration device between contractions to print at the 10 to 20 mm Hg line on the chart paper (see Figure 3-6)	8. To prevent missing the very beginning or ending of the uterine contraction, which is necessary for FHR pattern interpretation
9. Test the tocotransducer by applying slight pressure and observe the strip chart for a relative inflection of momentary increase from the "baseline"	9. To ensure that the transducer is pressure sensitive
10. Monitor the frequency and duration of the contractions and document them in the nurse's notes	10. The tocotransducer *cannot* measure intensity of contractions or resting tone between contractions because the depression of the pressure-sensing button varies with the amount of maternal adipose tissue; therefore the information should not be relied on to assess need for analgesia in relation to strength (painfulness) of contractions as registered by the monitor
11. When monitoring is in progress, readjust the abdominal strap periodically, and massage any reddened skin areas; a small amount of powder can be applied under the belt	11. To promote comfort and maintain the proper position of the transducer

Procedure	Rationale
12. Palpate the fundus every 15 to 30 minutes; *do not* rely on "peak pressure" of contraction to determine need for analgesia or titration of oxytocin	12. To assess relative pressure of contraction, because toco-transducer can relate only frequency and duration of contractions; it cannot assess intensity or resting tone
13. Reposition the transducer periodically and secure the abdominal belt snugly	13. To promote and ensure a good recording
14. When removing the toco-transducer, follow the procedure of the facility or follow the manufacturer's directions in the operating manual for cleaning and storage	14. To protect the surface of the transducer
15. Loosely coil the cable and secure with a rubber band, or place loosely coiled in a secure area	15. To prevent damage to the wires, which can occur with tight coiling
16. Dispose of disposable abdominal belt; wash reusable belt according to the facility's procedure before the next patient's use	16. To ensure that a disposable belt is not reused and that a reusable belt is cleaned and ready for future use

Advantages of the tocotransducer

- Noninvasive
- Does not require ruptured membranes or cervical dilatation
- Is easily applied
- May be used with telemetry

Limitations

- Information is limited to frequency and duration
- Cannot assess intensity of contractions
- Periodic repositioning of transducer may be necessary
- Limits patient's mobility
- May not get an interpretative tracing from an obese patient

Internal Mode of Monitoring
Spiral electrode

Description

The spiral electrode monitors the fetal ECG from the presenting part. It can be applied only after the membranes are ruptured, when the cervix is 2 to 3 cm or more dilated, and when the presenting part is accessible and identifiable (Figure 3-7). Therefore the spiral electrode can be used only during the intrapartum period. Use of the spiral electrode is contraindicated in patients suspected of having active herpes, group B streptococcus, HIV, or when there is undiagnosed vaginal bleeding (rule out placenta previa).

A sequential format for use of the spiral electrode is provided below.

Procedure	Rationale
1. Explain the procedure to the patient and her family	1. To allay anxiety
2. Gather necessary equipment: fetal monitor, disposable spiral electrode, leg plate with cable, leg plate strap, and electrode paste	2. To ensure that all equipment is readily accessible

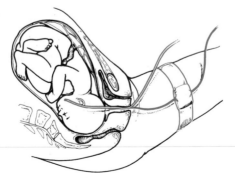

Figure 3-7
Diagrammatic representation of internal mode of monitoring with intrauterine catheter and spiral electrode in place.

Procedure	Rationale
3. Position the leg plate strap around the woman's thigh, securing the leg plate to the thigh	3. To ensure transmission of electrical signal
4. Insert the cable into the appropriate monitor connector labeled "ECG" or "cardio"	4. To connect cable plug to appropriate outlet
5. Assist the physician or nurse in performing a sterile vaginal examination in order to apply the spiral electrode a. Insert the entire apparatus through the vagina and cervix against the fetal presenting part b. Rotate the inner tube clockwise one full turn c. Remove and discard the outer drive tube	5. The electrode must be securely attached to ensure a good signal; the fetal face, fontanels, and genitals are avoided, and the electrode penetrates the skin of the presenting part 1.5 mm
6. Attach the disposable leg plate or the wires to the posts on the reusable leg plate	6. To provide proper polarity for ECG tracing
7. Turn on the power and observe the indicator light	7. To allow time for the monitor to process
8. Set the recorder at 3 cm/min paper speed, and observe the FHR on the strip chart	8. To ensure that the paper feeds correctly and that the recording is clear
9. Depress the test button for 10 seconds and make a notation of this on the strip chart; ensure that the monitor clock reflects the accurate time	9. To ensure that the monitor prints out a predetermined number (usually 120 or 150 bpm) on the corresponding line of the chart paper according to the manufacturer's guidelines in the operating manual
10. During monitoring check the leg plate periodically, and reposition for comfort as needed	10. To ensure transmission of the signal

Procedure	Rationale
NOTE: The spiral electrode must be moist in vaginal secretions or signal transmission may be impaired	
11. When removing the spiral electrode, turn 1½ turns counterclockwise or until it is free from the fetal presenting part; do not pull the electrode from the fetal skin; disconnect the electrode from the leg plate NOTE: The electrode should be removed just before cesarean delivery and should not be left attached and brought up through the uterine incision. If unable to detach, cut wire at perineum and notify physician	11. To ensure that the electrode is removed in the same manner that it is applied; pulling the electrode straight out results in unnecessary trauma to the fetal skin, produces an observable wound, and predisposes the site to infection
12. Remove the leg strap and dispose of it, if it is disposable, or wash if it is reusable	12. To ensure that the disposable belt is not reused and that the reusable belt is cleaned and ready for future use
13. Clean the reusable leg plate according to the facility's procedure, or follow the manufacturer's directions in the operating manual	13. To prevent infection
14. Loosely coil the cable and secure with a rubber band, or place loosely coiled in a secure area	14. To prevent damage to the wires, which can occur with tight coiling, resulting in loss of or an inadequate fetal signal
15. Clean the fetal insertion site with a povidone-iodine swab unless otherwise directed by hospital policy or procedure	15. To prevent infection

Advantages of the spiral electrode

- Can assess both long- and short-term variability
- Positional changes do not affect quality of tracing
- Can accurately display fetal cardiac dysrhythmias
- Accurately displays FHR between 30 and 240 bpm

Limitations

- Membranes must be ruptured
- Cervix must be dilated at least 2 cm
- Presenting part must be accessible
- Need moist environment for FHR detection (difficult to monitor when fetal head is crowning)
- May record maternal heart rate (with fetal demise)
- May miss fetal dysrhythmias if logic or ECG activation switch is engaged

Intrauterine (transcervical) catheter

Description

The intrauterine catheter monitors contraction frequency, duration, intensity, and resting tone. A small catheter is introduced vaginally (transcervically) into the uterus after the cervix is dilated 2 to 3 cm and the fetal membranes have been ruptured. The catheter is compressed during uterine contractions, placing pressure on a strain gauge, or pressure transducer. The pressure is then reflected on the strip chart in the form of mm Hg pressure (Figure 3-8).

Some internal pressure catheters have the pressure-sensing device within the catheter tip. These do not require the instillation of sterile water for use. Some of the newer catheters are provided with a double lumen (Intran Plus IUP-400) to allow simultaneous amniofusion and uterine activity monitoring.

Procedure	Rationale
1. Explain the procedure to the patient and her family	1. To allay anxiety
2. Gather necessary equipment: fetal monitor, disposable intrauterine kit, sterile gloves, and other equipment to perform a sterile vaginal examination	2. To ensure that all equipment is readily accessible

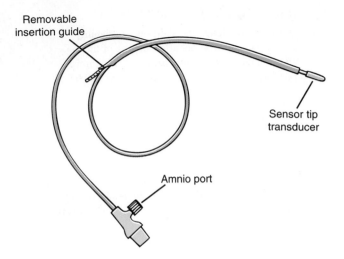

Figure 3-8
Intrauterine catheter with the sensor transducer located in the tip of the catheter provides uninterrupted uterine activity monitoring. Saline-filled catheters are another type of catheter in use. Note that this catheter has an amnioport that may be used for an amnioinfusion.

Procedure	Rationale
3. Insert the reusable cable into the appropriate monitor connector labeled "uterine activity," "toco," or "utero"	3. To activate the pressure transducer
4. Before inserting a "fluid-filled catheter," fill the catheter with 5 ml sterile water, leaving the syringe attached to the catheter; maintain sterility of the maternal end of the catheter	4. To ensure that the catheter is patent and fluid-filled before insertion; to maintain aseptic technique
5. Prepare the patient for a sterile vaginal examination; the examining fingers are placed just inside the cervix	5. To maintain aseptic technique and to identify the location for catheter insertion

Procedure	Rationale
6. Insert the sterile catheter within the catheter guide no more than 2 cm inside the cervix	6. The guide is made of a very hard plastic that can cause trauma if inserted farther than necessary
7. Advance the catheter according to the insertion depth indicator or until the blue or black mark on it reaches the vaginal introitus	7. To ensure that enough of the catheter is inside the uterus
8. Slide the catheter guide away from the introitus and remove it from the opposite end (or after cleaning the guide, tape it securely over the top or across the side of the monitor)	8. To prevent the guide from sliding toward the introitus
9. Tape the catheter securely to the patient's leg	9. To ensure patient mobility without fear of dislodging the catheter
10. Connect the intrauterine transducer-tipped catheter to the cable and zero it by turning the pressure knob to ensure that the pen reads/prints at the zero line of the strip chart, or connect the fluid-filled catheter to the strain gauge apparatus (pressure transducer) via the three-way stopcock	10. To ensure appropriate location of strain gauge in relation to the uterus

Perform the following procedures only for fluid-filled catheters:

a. Test or calibrate the strain gauge according to the manufacturer's instructions	a. To validate that uterine activity information is correct
b. Keeping the stopcock "Off" position pointed to the strain gauge, flush the catheter with 5 ml sterile water	b. To ensure that the catheter is patent and completely filled with fluid

Procedure	Rationale
c. Rotate the stopcock lever so that the "Off" position points to the catheter	c. To exclude pressure to the strain gauge
d. Release the pressure valve on the strain gauge and inject water from the syringe through the stopcock and gauge until all air bubbles are removed	d. To ensure that the strain gauge is completely filled with fluid
e. Release the pressure relief valve and then remove the syringe from the stopcock, maintaining its sterility	e. To open the system to atmospheric pressure
f. Turn on the power and press the record button; observe the tracing, which should print on the zero line of the uterine activity section of the chart paper; turn the pressure knob to ensure that the pen reads just at the zero line of the chart paper; (do not turn it to go below zero)	f. To verify that the tracing prints out on the zero line in the absence of pressure
g. Depress the test button for 10 seconds and make a notation of this on the tracing; the monitor will print a predetermined number, usually at the 50 mm Hg line of the chart paper, according to the manufacturer's operating manual; if it does not read 50 mm Hg, adjust the pressure knob to ensure that the pen points at the zero line of the chart paper and then test it again (Figure 3-9)	g. To ensure that the monitor traces on the appropriate line; this validates the accuracy of subsequent internal pressure monitoring

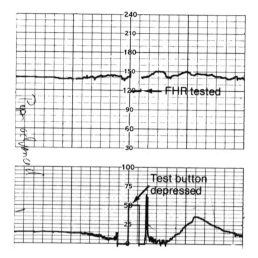

Figure 3-9
FHR and uterine activity tested for the internal mode of monitoring.

Procedure	Rationale
h. Reattach the syringe to the stopcock; rotate the stopcock lever so that the "Off" position is pointing to the syringe; the uterine pressure system is now ready for monitoring	h. The solid column of water places pressure on the diaphragm of the strain gauge when it is compressed by uterine contractions; this results in an inflection on the uterine activity section of the strip chart in mm Hg
i. When monitoring is in progress:	
(1) Flush the intrauterine catheter with sterile water every 2 hours or as necessary (the use of solutions other than sterile water can occlude and corrode the system)	(1) To remove any vernix caseosa or air bubbles that may have entered the catheter and can invalidate the pressure reading

Procedure	Rationale
(2) Check the proper functioning of the catheter when necessary by tapping the catheter, asking the patient to cough, or applying fundal pressure while observing the chart	(2) To ensure inflection on the chart paper
11. Zero the catheter and test according to the manufacturer's directions	11. To ensure that the monitor traces on the appropriate line; this validates the accuracy of subsequent internal pressure monitoring
12. Apply gentle traction to remove catheter and dispose of catheter appropriately	12. To ensure that disposable equipment is not reused

Advantages of the intrauterine catheter

- Less confining and more comfortable than external mode of uterine activity monitoring
- Only accurate measure of uterine activity (e.g., frequency, duration, intensity, and resting tone)
- May be used with telemetry
- Records accurately regardless of maternal position

Limitations

- Membranes must be ruptured and cervix sufficiently dilated (e.g., 2 to 3 cm)
- Improper insertion can cause maternal trauma
- Increased risk of infection

Troubleshooting the Monitor

The electronic fetal monitor is a useful tool to assess fetal well-being. As with any electronic device, problems may occur that can often be overcome. The following section suggests actions for identified problems.

Problem	Action
Power	■ Check power cord at wall and back of monitor
	■ Push in both ends of cord to ensure a tight fit (it may appear intact, although it is not)
Sixty-cycle interference	■ Check FHR by auscultation
	■ If there is improper grounding at the outlet, plug, or in machine, change to another electrical outlet, switch cords, or change electrode wires (on ground cable)
	■ Change electrode or monitor
Ultrasound *Half or double rate*	■ Check with fetoscope, stethoscope, or Doppler
	■ Check maternal pulse to rule out maternal signal and document maternal pulse
	■ Consider applying spiral electrode, or call physician to apply electrode if membranes are intact and bradycardia is present
	■ Add coupling gel and recheck
	■ Move transducer to search for a better signal
Intermittent ultrasound signal	■ Check ultrasound transducer: hold transducer by cord, allow transducer to hang, turn up volume, swing ultrasound transducer in the air; if static is heard, replace transducer; apply label to broken transducer for repair or replacement
	■ Check cable insertion site for a tight fit
Intermittent or no signal	■ Check gel on transducer; it may be dry (when gel is dry, sound waves do not penetrate the skin); reapply gel; move transducer if fetus is out of range
Autocorrelation limitations	■ Verify FHR by auscultation. (Autocorrelation compares new data to last several beats; at times can exclude data from the comparison or can produce a false signal in the absence of fetal cardiac motion by enhancing signal-to-noise levels)

Problem	Action
Direct FHR monitoring with spiral electrode	
Intermittent signal (individual dots on monitor strip or no signal)	■ Do vaginal exam; check electrode placement; if loose, replace electrode
	■ Check that reference electrode is in vaginal secretions (instill fluid if necessary)
	■ Check ground cable on leg for adherence to skin
	■ If still no signal, remove red wire from ground cable, replace with disposable electrode and reference electrode wire
Signal and recording with stillborn (maternal signal is conducted through the stillborn infant)	■ Check and document maternal pulse (radial)
	■ Check with doptone and suggest ultrasound to check for heart motion
Tocodynamometer (toco)	
■ No recording	■ Readjust toco on patient
■ Numbers in high range	■ Turn down the setting to a lower number on toco channel (if numbers cannot be turned down, toco needs repair); replace with another toco
Toco not picking up contractions	■ Palpate abdomen for best quality of contractions and reapply toco
	■ Place elastic belts tighter, or use another device to hold toco firmly against abdomen
	■ Consider using intrauterine pressure catheter (IUPC) if patient is significantly obese
Intrauterine pressure catheter (IUPC)	
Not recording	■ Recheck cable insertion
Resting tone (6 to 15 mm Hg)	■ Adjust level of strain gauge for fluid-filled catheters
	■ Flush fluid-filled catheter
	■ Recalibrate nonfluid-filled catheter

Problem	Action
Not recording contractions	▪ Check catheter markings at patient's introitus (catheter may have slipped out)
	▪ Replace catheter if necessary
High resting tone	▪ Higher resting tone may be noted for: Pitocin (20 mm Hg) Twins (30 mm Hg) Amnionitis (30 to 40 mm Hg)

Other problems

Dysrhythmia (occurs in 5% of pregnancies)	▪ Turn up volume (can dysrhythmia be heard?)
	▪ Consult with other health professionals
	▪ Check for variability, tachycardia, and bradycardia
	▪ Perform fetal ECG
Errors caused by incorrect paper speed or monitor paper with different scale	▪ Check annotation with paper speed; it should be 3 cm/min
	▪ Check scale; it should be 30 to 240 bpm for FHR

Display of Fetal Heart Rate and Uterine Activity

FHR is recorded on the upper section of the chart paper, and uterine activity is recorded on the lower section (Figure 3-10). The FHR is printed on a vertical scale with a range of 30 to 240 bpm. The horizontal scale is divided into 1-minute sections, which are subdivided by six sections representing 10 seconds each.

The lower section is used to record uterine activity. The vertical scale ranges from 0 to 100 mm Hg pressure and is accurate in assessing intensity of contractions only when the intrauterine catheter is used. The horizontal scale represents time as previously described. The lower section of the chart paper can be used to assess frequency of contractions, usually measured from peak to peak (or from onset of one uterine contraction to the onset of the next uterine contraction), and duration of contractions. Because the inflections of uterine activity, which are noted on the chart paper and assessed with the tocotransducer, are dependent on the thickness of maternal adipose tissue and tocotransducer placement over the maternal uterine fundus, it must be remembered that the intensity of uterine contractions cannot be assessed by use of the external mode of monitoring.

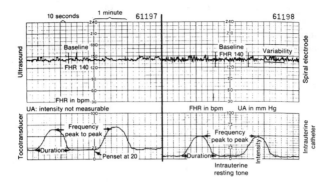

Figure 3-10

Display of FHR and uterine activity on monitor strip.
A, External mode of monitoring with ultrasound and
tocotransducer. **B,** Internal mode of monitoring with spiral
electrode and intrauterine catheter. Other significant
information is supplied.

Telemetry

Remote internal or external FHR monitoring via radio wave telemetry (Figure 3-11) helps patients to remain ambulatory without the
loss of continuous monitoring data. The patient may feel less con-
fined, more relaxed, and more content if she can walk around. The
transducer is worn by the patient by means of a shoulder strap or
other device (Figure 3-12). Heart rate and uterine activity signals
are continuously transmitted to a receiver that is connected to the fetal monitor. The monitor then processes the data, displays, and prints
the heart rate and uterine activity on the strip chart. The fetal monitor receiving data should be connected to a central display or should
be located to ensure surveillance by clinicians.

In addition to the benefits of freedom of movement during labor
and continuous monitoring during transport within the labor suite
or to the delivery room, telemetry has been applied in the outpatient
setting for patients instructed to remain at rest in their own homes.

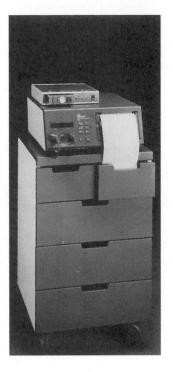

Figure 3-11
Telemetry unit on top of fetal monitor.
(Courtesy Corometrics Medical Systems, Inc., Wallingford, Conn.)

Data from the transmitter can be sent via modem to the receiver unit, which is connected to a printer, producing a hard copy of the FHR strip chart. This transmission of information from the patient to the receiver unit allows the clinician to determine the patient's status. Based on the data received, the patient's tocolytic needs may be adjusted, and consultation can be made with a referral center by the clinician to receive an expert's interpretation of the data.

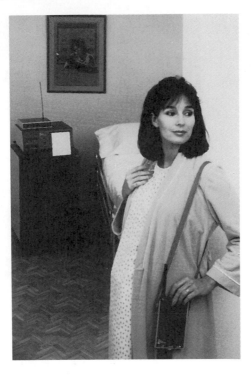

Figure 3-12
Ambulatory patient being monitored with telemetry unit.
(Courtesy Corometrics Medical Systems, Inc., Wallingford, Conn.)

Central Display

A central monitor display at the nurses' station provides an opportunity to view tracings from several patients at the same time (Figure 3-13). In addition, single screen display of several patients can
be accessed from remote locations including the patient's bedside,
staff locker room or lounge areas, or a physician's office. This can
provide the staff with instant access to the patient's monitor pattern
from any location and is especially important when the nurse cannot
be in constant attendance. Some systems include the capability of
data entry in the form of detailed notes about results of examinations, cervical dilatation, fetal station, administration of drugs, pa-

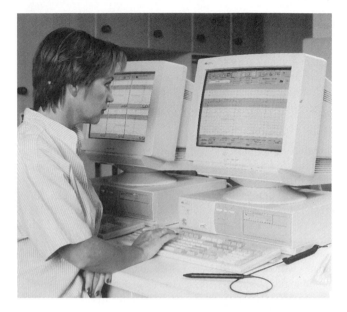

Figure 3-13
At the central station there is an instant overview of every
patient monitored. HP *OB TraceVue* provides obstetrical
surveillance with alerts for fetal tachycardia/bradycardia, signal
loss, coincidental fetal and maternal heart rates, and other
parameters at the bedside, central station, or at remote
office/home site. It can be connected to both HP and non-HP
fetal monitors. Optional trace storage to an optical laser disk
permits archiving of thousands of fetal traces.
(Courtesy Hewlett-Packard, Böblingen, Germany.)

tient's position, and vital signs, all related to time. Reports may be
generated with the integration of an optional printer linked to the
display, which can contain complete patient information, history,
and a graphic printout of the labor curve progression, providing a
single and comprehensive document.

Some central display systems can provide additional information, including the following:
1. A system status screen provides an instant overview of several beds
   on the system and indicates any alerts by room number. In addition,
   it can identify the signal source of any of the patients on the system.

2. A trend screen, which can provide the most recent past few minutes of heart rate and uterine activity data on any one patient,
with immediate warning of critical conditions relating to any patient in the system.
3. An alert screen, which provides an immediate summary of the
trend analysis on any patient. The data can be made available to
the staff before, during, and after an alert.

Archival and Retrieval

Traditional long-term storage of fetal monitoring strips has been
problematic for most medical record units in terms of time and
space. Microfiche records of the strip chart are less bulky to store
but still take time to log, sort, and file in the medical record. An alternative to this is the capability of new central monitoring systems
that store patient information and data from the monitors, including direct intrapartum and antepartum recordings. The data are
stored by the central computer on hard drives or floppy disks. Some
systems with optical disk storage hold approximately 28,000 hours
of monitor data, which is enough for about 3000 patients. The ability to record, store, retrieve, and reproduce the tracing is a significant advance in the archiving and retrieval of fetal monitoring data.

Data Input Devices

Data input devices are now an option with some electronic fetal
monitors and monitoring systems. Some of the options include use
of a barcode reader, key pads for data entry (Figure 3-14), light pens
(Figure 3-15), and standard keyboards. The input is subsequently
printed on the strip chart (Figure 3-16). The use of these options can
promote accurate documentation and help to eliminate the need for
handwritten annotations, which are sometimes illegible. In addition,
some information may be entered on the strip chart automatically,
including time (every 10 minutes), date, chart speed, monitoring,
and baseline pressure off scale.

Artifact Detection

Fetal monitors have built-in artifact rejection systems, which are always in operation when using the external mode of FHR monitoring.
Logic circuitry rejects data when there is a greater variation than is

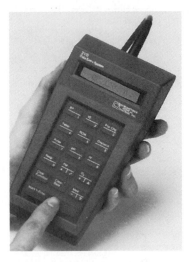

Figure 3-14
Data entry keypad helps to eliminate the need for handwritten annotations and can be used at the patient's bedside.
(Courtesy Corometrics Medical Systems, Inc., Wallingford, Conn.)

expected between successive fetal heartbeats. If there are repetitive variations by more than the accepted amount, the older generation monitors may switch from a hold mode to a nonrecord mode (exhibited by penlift or no heat to the stylus). The recorder resumes recording when the variation between successive beats falls within the predetermined parameters. The newer monitors continue to print regardless of the extent of the excursion of the fetal heart rate.

During internal monitoring, artifact is rare, and the logic system will miss only those changes that exceed the predetermined limits of the system. If there is an accessible switch to select a logic or no-logic mode, it is preferable to have the monitor in the no-logic mode when using the internal mode (spiral electrode) in order to detect fetal arrhythmias. When recording internally, the logic-on should

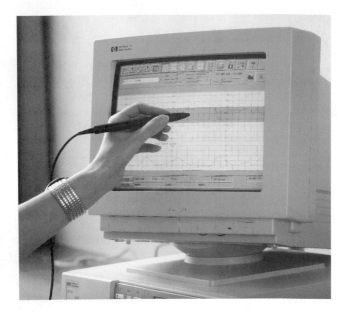

Figure 3-15
With color icons one can enter and access information quickly and easily with a light pen, mouse, or keyboard.
(Courtesy Hewlett-Packard, Böblingen, Germany.)

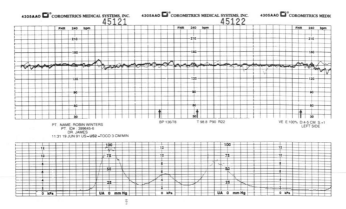

Figure 3-16
Tracing demonstrates pertinent data that has been entered via a data input device.
(Courtesy Corometrics Medical Systems, Inc., Wallingford, Conn.)

be used only when there is true artifact, such as with poor signal-to-noise ratio (caused by extraneous electrical noise), or when there is a large maternal R wave that is counted on an intermittent basis. This can usually be determined by printing out the fetal ECG.

Considerations Before Monitor Purchase

Various monitors are available, and generally they have the same capabilities. In considering a monitor for purchase, however, it is prudent to use the desired model on a trial basis and to consult with people who have used the type of equipment being considered (Figures 3-17, 3-18, and 3-19). The following items should also be considered:

1. Accuracy of data output
2. Ease of use

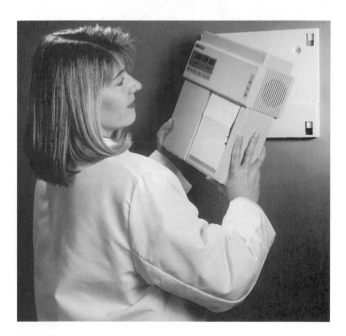

Figure 3-17
Space-saving designed HP Series 50 A and IP fetal monitors are compact, lightweight, and function equally well mounted on a wall, tabletop, or mobile cart.
(Courtesy Hewlett-Packard, Böblingen, Germany.)

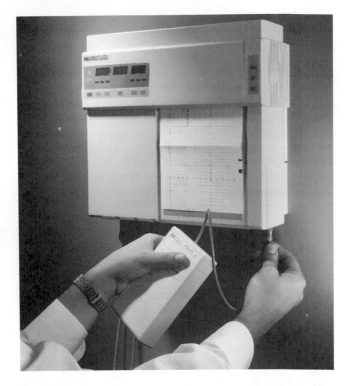

Figure 3-18
An upgrade key assures the addition of new features and future developments, thus protecting the initial investment for years to come.
(Courtesy Hewlett-Packard, Böblingen, Germany.)

3. Reliability for continuous functioning with minimum down/re-pair time
4. Repair frequency and history from other facilities using the same monitor (turnaround time for service)
5. Cost of monitor and other expendable supplies (e.g., paper, ab-dominal belts)
6. Availability of expendable supplies from multiple sources for better cost advantage

7. Legible display and function labels
8. Complexity of paper refill procedure
9. Training time needed for users or video training films included with purchase
10. Fragility of ultrasound transducer, cable, and connectors
11. History and stability of company and frequency of changing models
12. Expected life of the equipment
13. Interchangeability of transducers from one model to the next within the same company (to avoid the possibility of built-in obsolescence)

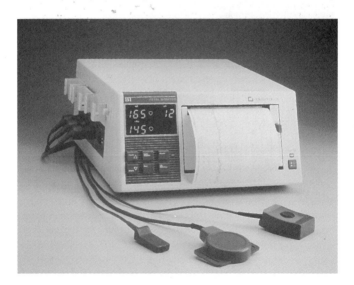

Figure 3-19

Corometrics Model 151 fetal monitor provides internal and external monitoring, twin monitoring, documentation (time, date, mode of monitoring, and paper speed are printed on strip chart), and connects to a noninvasive blood pressure monitor and to a data entry keyboard for the annotation of clinical notes.

(Courtesy Corometrics Medical Systems, Inc., Wallingford, Conn.)

Uterine Activity Monitoring

4

One of the benefits of electronic FHR monitoring is the data provided about uterine activity. Frequency, duration, and strength of uterine contractions can be determined by manual palpation, but the absolute intensity of the contractions cannot be measured in this manner. In addition to quantifying intensity of contractions via the intrauterine catheter, the monitor provides a permanent record of uterine activity.

Uterine activity is monitored on the lower section of the chart panel. Each major vertical division represents 25 mm Hg pressure, with the smaller lines representing 5 mm Hg. There are major differences between the external mode of monitoring and the internal mode in terms of obtainable uterine activity data. The following list contrasts these two modes of monitoring.

	External Mode	Internal Mode
Signal source	Tocotransducer (tocodynamometer)	Intrauterine (transcervical) catheter
Data	1. Frequency of contractions (measured from the onset of one contraction to the onset of the next contraction)	1. Frequency of contractions (measured from peak to peak or from the onset of one contraction to the onset of the next contraction)
	2. Duration of contractions (from beginning to end)	2. Duration of contractions (from beginning to end)

External Mode	Internal Mode
3. Relative strength of contractions; inflection on UA panel of chart paper is made by the contraction of the uterus, which depresses a pressure-sensing button (a thin patient may exhibit large inflections when having only mild contractions; in contrast, an obese patient may exhibit minor inflections when having strong contractions; the nurse must then palpate the abdomen to assess relative strength of contraction and degree of indentation of the fundus)	3. Intensity of contractions (mm Hg pressure at peak of contraction) 4. Resting tone (mm Hg pressure between contractions)

It is important to note that belt tightness, position of the tocodynamometer, and maternal position can all greatly affect the recording of uterine activity. In addition, the toco reflects only relative strength of a contraction, which must be assessed by palpation. The toco cannot assess intensity of uterine contractions.

In a normal labor, uterine contractions occur about every 3 to 5 minutes, with a duration of 30 to 60 seconds, an intensity of 50 to 75 mm Hg, and a resting tone between 5 and 15 mm Hg. In addition to identifying this information, the chart panel also indicates fetal movement by "blips," spikes, or momentary increases in uterine pressure. Identification of fetal movement is important, as it forms the basis for antepartum nonstress testing by identifying fetal reactivity or the presence of accelerations with fetal movement.

During intrapartum monitoring it is important to look for hyperstimulation of the uterus in addition to the frequency, duration, and intensity of contractions and uterine resting tone. Hyperstimulation, as evidenced by increased uterine activity on the chart panel, can result in an asphyxiated fetus (because of interference with the placental circulation) and potentially in uterine rupture. An outlined description of increased uterine activity follows.

Increased Uterine Activity

Observations

1. Contractions lasting longer than 90 seconds
2. Relaxation between contractions less than 30 seconds
3. Inadequate intrauterine relaxation with resting tone above 15 mm Hg between contractions
4. Peak pressure of contractions above 80 mm Hg
5. Contractions more frequent than every 2 minutes

Causes

1. Hyperstimulation of the uterus with oxytocin
2. Abruptio placentae
3. Overdistension of the uterine wall as a result of multiple gestation, hydramnios, or a macrosomic fetus
4. Pregnancy-induced hypertension
5. Drugs
   a. Narcotics (e.g., meperidine hydrochloride [Demerol])
   b. Catecholamines (adrenergics) (e.g., norepinephrine [Noradrenaline, Levarterenol])
   c. Beta-blocking agents (e.g., propranolol [Inderal])
   d. Prostaglandins (e.g., prostaglandin E_2 alpha [$PGE_2\alpha$, Dinoprost])
   e. Pituitary hormones (e.g., vasopressin [Pitressin])
   f. Quinine
   g. Estrogen
   h. Ergonovine
   i. Acetylcholine

Clinical Significance

Hyperstimulation of the uterus or hypertonus can result in stress to the fetus (as a result of the lack of placental perfusion) and potentially in uterine rupture. The most common cause of uterine hyperstimulation is the injudicious use of oxytocin. When an oxytocin infusion is discontinued, uterine relaxation usually occurs within 10 minutes with return of normal baseline FHR and variability. When oxytocin is given by poorly controlled methods, such as the buccal or intramuscular route, there is an added risk because the rate of absorption, as well as any adverse fetal effects, is prolonged

(Figure 4-1). A protocol for the administration of oxytocin for induction or augmentation of labor is in Appendix B.

Because uterine contractions are known to decrease the rate of blood flow through the intervillous space and most fetuses are well able to tolerate this transient type of stress, it is important for the nurse to attentively monitor uterine activity in addition to FHR. In pregnancies in which the margin of fetal reserve is low, this phenomenon can cause commensurate decreases in FHR (described as late decelerations). The physician should be promptly notified when there is evidence of uterine hyperstimulation with or without an associated heart rate response.

Intervention

1. Discontinue oxytocin if infusing (exercise caution in flushing the oxytocin out of the line to ensure that a bolus is not delivered to the patient).
2. Increase rate of maintenance intravenous infusion.
3. Change maternal position (left lateral preferred).
4. Consider administration of oxygen, 8 to 12 L/min by face mask, depending on response in FHR.
5. The physician may consider the use of tocolytics such as terbutaline, magnesium sulfate, or ritodrine if there is an excessive increase in uterine activity, such as hypertonus, and a nonreassuring FHR pattern is evident.

Fetal recovery from uterine hypertonus is preferred in utero because once the placental circulation is restored, carbon dioxide from

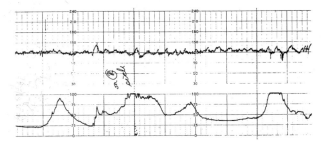

Figure 4-1
Uterine hyperstimulation from oxytocin.

respiratory acidosis, as well as the acidic products of anaerobic metabolism, can be eliminated.

Inhibition of Uterine Activity
Tocolytics

It is important to decrease uterine activity when premature labor or nonreassuring FHR patterns occur. Drugs such as isoxsuprine, epinephrine, and isoproterenol have been used in the past to reduce uterine activity but not without drawbacks (i.e., their beta-stimulant effects cause vasodilation and secondary hypotension). Because of their extrauterine effects, beta-mimetic agents are now used. Terbutaline is now routinely used because it has maximal uterine relaxant effects. In addition, nifedipine is frequently considered as the first choice in tocolytic therapy. Other drugs known to inhibit uterine activity include diazoxide, halothane, progesterone, and prostaglandin inhibitors (e.g., ibuprofen and indomethacin).

In the past alcohol was widely used to successfully stop premature labor in some patients, but in others it had detrimental results. It is no longer used, however. Alcohol can depress maternal central respiratory and vasomotor centers, inducing secondary hypoxia.

See the box for a list of drugs known to inhibit uterine activity. A protocol for the management of preterm labor can be found in Appendix C.

Drugs Inhibiting Uterine Activity

1. Beta-sympathomimetics (e.g., terbutaline and ritodrine)
2. Calcium-channel blocker (e.g., nifedipine)
3. Prostaglandin inhibitors (e.g., indomethacin)
4. Magnesium sulfate
5. Diazoxide
6. Ethanol
7. Halothane
8. Progesterone

Baseline Fetal Heart Rate

5

Since the advent and wide acceptance of electronic fetal monitoring (EFM), a variety of classification methods has been used to describe all aspects of the fetal heart rate. These methods vary widely from institution to institution and from practitioner to practitioner. Because of this variation in interpretation of EFM and, to date, the lack of consistently accepted definitions for EFM terms, it is expected that each member of the health care team caring for the intrapartum patient on EFM will agree on what objective criteria will be used when interpreting EFM tracings in their institution. It is recommended that all members of the obstetrical nursing and medical team meet and concur on standards and definitions that will define FHR interpretation and EFM practice in their institution. This then becomes the institution-specific policy and procedure. In the event that consensus cannot be reached between medical and nursing staff, "it is reasonable for the department of obstetric nursing to set forth objective criteria based on EFM literature to be used consistently by nursing staff" (Miller, 1994).

Baseline FHR is the intrinsic rhythm of the fetal heart. Evaluation of baseline FHR occurs over a 10- to 20-minute time frame. The definition of baseline FHR (Figure 5-1) is that heart rate that occurs when there is no stress on or stimulation to the fetus, for example:

1. When the patient is not in labor
2. When the fetus is not moving
3. Between uterine contractions
4. When there is no stimulation to the fetus as occurs with vaginal examinations and electrode application
5. During the interval between periodic changes

Baseline FHR is set by the atrial pacemaker and balanced by an interplay between the sympathetic (cardioaccelerator) and parasympathetic (decelerator) branches of the autonomic nervous system. As a result of immaturity of the central nervous system and the sympathetic dominance, the premature fetus at approximately 20 weeks

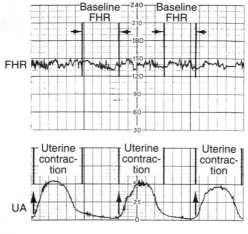

Figure 5-1
Baseline fetal heart rate is identified between uterine contractions.

gestation may exhibit a baseline heart rate of 160 bpm. In the healthy full-term infant, the rate is usually between 120 and 160 bpm. This is the result of the balanced regulatory interaction between parasympathetic and sympathetic nervous systems. A fetus over the age of 40 weeks gestation may have a rate between 110 and 120 bpm. This rate indicates a slightly greater influence of parasympathetic control.

Variability

Description

Variability of the FHR can be described as the normal irregularity of cardiac rhythm, resulting from a continuous balancing interaction of the sympathetic (cardioacceleration) and parasympathetic (cardiodeceleration) branches of the autonomic nervous system. These two branches interact, modulating the FHR. Average variability of the FHR is demonstrated by fluctuations of the baseline, which reflect an intact neurological pathway, optimal fetal oxygenation, and the measure of fetal oxygen reserve in the tissue. In addition, intrapartum baseline variability indirectly indicates fetal tolerance of labor.

Variability is considered to be the most important FHR characteristic and reflects appropriate neurological modulation of the FHR. The fetus who exhibits normal or average variability (reassuring) indicates a capability to centralize available oxygen and will remain physiologically compensated. If each interval between successive heartbeats were exactly the same, as in the regular rhythm of a ticking clock or metronome, the baseline would be flat, indicating central nervous system depression associated with hypoxia. Therefore, absence of variability of the FHR is demonstrated by a smooth or flat baseline.

The normal irregularity is further described as *short-term variability (STV)* or *long-term variability (LTV)*. STV (beat-to-beat) is described as the internal difference between successive R peaks of the fetal electrocardiogram (FECG) signal (Figure 5-2). It is a reflection of the normal irregularity in the interval between consecu-

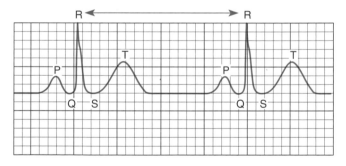

Figure 5-2

Fetal heart rate tracings from a fetal spiral electrode are obtained by FECG measuring the interval between consecutive fetal R waves. A cardiotachometer processes the interval between R waves to a rate in beats per minute, which is printed on the monitoring tracing. This illustration demonstrates the time interval between R waves. However, in the healthy fetus the intervals should vary, showing variability in the fetal heart rate.

tive heartbeats (cardiac rhythm) and is controlled by the parasympathetic nervous system. Direct ECG (scalp electrode) is the only method that can accurately measure STV (Freeman, Garite, and Nageotte, 1991). STV is the sensitive indicator of fetal oxygenation and oxygen reserve in the tissue. Presence of STV is reassuring in that it indicates that the fetus appropriately responds to nerve impulses and has an intact autonomic nervous system. Literature and practice vary on labels placed on STV: present or absent (AWHONN, 1993); or absent, decreased, average, or increased (Afriat, 1989). This is an example of the need for a consensus on the institution-specific definition of FHR interpretation.

LTV is the rhythmic fluctuations or cyclic variations of 6 to 10 bpm in amplitude around FHR baseline in 3 to 10 cycles per minute. It is evaluated over 5 to 10 minutes of a FHR tracing (Table 5-1). LTV is measured between contractions and periodic changes and excludes any aberrant marks and artifact. Interpretation of LTV is made by visual examination of the amplitude and frequency of changes or waves in the baseline. It is a marker for fetal hypoxia that requires intervention and is an interpretative guideline that gives an indication of fetal oxygenation and physiologic ability to compensate for stress. The sympathetic nervous system influences LTV.

Table 5-1   Fetal heart rate variability

	Short Term	Long Term
Description	A change in FHR from one beat to the next "beat-to-beat"	Rhythmic and cyclic fluctuations in FHR of 3 to 10 cycles per minute
Appearance		
Signal source	Spiral electrode	Internal and external modes of monitoring

Generally, short- and long-term variability tend to increase and decrease together. This is caused by the interplay between the parasympathetic and sympathetic nervous system and their response to external and internal factors. There are also certain instances when STV and LTV exhibit changes independently from each other (Figure 5-3). When evaluating STV and LTV, the effect of factors such as gestational age, drugs, stage of labor, anesthesia, maternal risk history, and fetal anomalies and condition have to be considered when making a determination of whether variability is reassuring or nonreassuring. A decision to intervene may follow this determination.

Literature and practice vary on labels placed on LTV. Classifications range from 5 categories to 2. Five categories for LTV classification (Figure 5-4) are: absent, minimal, average, moderate, and marked (Murray, 1988; Parer, 1983). Other categories for LTV classification are: present and decreased (Afriat, 1989); decreased or minimal (0 to 5 bpm), average or within normal limits (6 to 25 bpm), or marked or saltatory (>25 bpm) (AWHONN, 1993). This is an example of the need for a consensus on the institution-specific definition of FHR interpretation in order to guide practice.

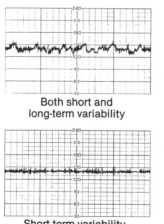

Both short and
long-term variability

Short-term variability,
absence of long-term variability

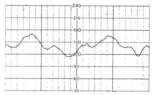

Long-term variability,
absence of short-term variability

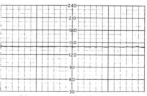

Absence of both short
and long-term variability

Figure 5-3
Variations in short- and long-term variability.

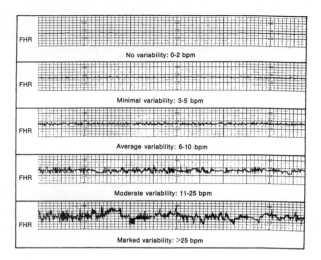

Figure 5-4
Classification of long-term variability.

External ultrasound most accurately demonstrates long-term variability but inconsistently demonstrates short-term variability because of limitations encountered during monitoring, including maternal and fetal coincidental heartbeats, movement, and maternal muscle activity.

Variations in Variability

Appearance and Cause	Clinical Significance/Intervention
1. Mild hypoxia ($\uparrow$STV) An early compensatory mechanism produces an increase in FHR variability	The significance of marked variability is not known. Increased variability from a previous average variability is thought to be a compensatory mechanism and an early sign of fetal hypoxia. Unless deterioration of variability or a nonreassuring pattern develops, no intervention is required. Efforts to improve and enhance fetal oxygenation and uteroplacental bloodflow through maternal positioning, hydration, correction of ma-
2. Fetal stimulation ($\uparrow$STV, LTV) External uterine palpation, uterine contractions, fetal activity, application of spiral electrode, vaginal examination,	

acoustic stimulation, and maternal activity stimulate the fetal autonomic nervous system, resulting in an increase in variability

3. Illicit Drugs (↑STV, LTV)
   Initial response is central nervous system (CNS) excitability to cocaine and methamphetamines

4. Hypoxia and acidosis (↓STV, LTV)
   Uteroplacental insufficiency as a result of several causes (uterine hyperstimulation, maternal supine hypotension, pregnancy-induced hypertension, amnionitis). (Other causes are listed under late decelerations.)

ternal hypotension, maternal oxygenation, and eliminating uterine hyperstimulation are indicated.

Decreasing variability is a warning of fetal stress. Absence of variability exhibited by a smooth or flat baseline is a significant sign of fetal distress. A flat or smooth baseline associated with late decelerations of *any* magnitude is a sign of advanced hypoxia and acidosis that is related to central nervous system depression. Decreased variability related to drugs usually returns to previous baseline levels as the drug is excreted. If a CNS-depressant drug has been given and delivery appears imminent, Narcan may be administered to the mother just before delivery or to the neonate after delivery. Baseline variability should be evaluated before administration of analgesics/narcotics and administration time and effect documented. Variability that is decreased as a result of fetal sleep patterns usually resumes in 20 to 30 minutes. Efforts to improve and enhance fetal oxygenation and uteroplacental bloodflow through maternal positioning, hydration, correction of maternal hypotension, maternal oxygenation, and eliminating uterine hyperstimulation are indicated. Applica-

Variations in Variability

Appearance and Cause	Clinical Significance/Intervention
	tion of a spiral electrode should be considered if the pattern is observed by external monitoring.
5. Drugs (↓STV, ↓LTV) Narcotics, tranquilizers, barbiturates, and anesthetics depress central nervous system mechanisms responsible for cardiac control; anticholinergics such as atropine and scopolamine block the transmission of impulses to the sinoatrial node *Analgesics/narcotics* Meperidine hydrochloride (Demerol), morphine sulfate, nalbuphine hydrochloride (Nubain), butorphanol tartrate (Stadol), sublimaze (Fentanyl) *Barbiturates* Secobarbital sodium (Seconal), pentobarbital sodium (Nembutal), amobarbital (Amytal) *Tranquilizers* Diazepam (Valium) *Phenothiazines* Promethazine hydrochloride (Phenergan), propiomazine hydrochloride (Largon), hydroxyzine pamoate (Vistaril), promazine hydrochloride (Sparine) *Parasympatholytics* Atropine *General anesthetics*	Baseline variability should be evaluated before administration of analgesics/narcotics and administration time and effect documented. Efforts to improve and enhance fetal oxygenation and uteroplacental bloodflow through maternal positioning, hydration, correction of maternal hypotension, maternal oxygenation, and eliminating uterine hyperstimulation are indicated. Application of a spiral electrode should be considered if the pattern is observed by external monitoring.

Variations in Variability Appearance and Cause	Clinical Significance/Intervention
6. Fetal sleep cycles (↓LTV) Periods of fetal sleep, usually lasting for 20 to 30 minutes, produce decreased long-term variability; does not usually affect short-term variability	Variability that is decreased as a result of fetal sleep patterns usually resumes in 20 to 30 minutes.
7. Congenital anomalies (↓STV, ↓LTV) Central nervous system (e.g., anencephaly) or cardiac anomalies can decrease variability	No intervention can reverse congenital anomalies or extreme prematurity.
8. Fetal cardiac dysrhythmias (↓STV, ↓LTV) Suppression of cardiac control mechanisms may be the result of paroxysmal atrial tachycardia, complete heart block, nodal rhythm, or an aberrant pacemaker	Some cardiac drugs may be given via the mother in an attempt to cardiovert some dysrhythmias.
9. Extreme prematurity (<24 weeks) (↓LTV) Heartbeat is controlled by immature neurological mechanisms, resulting in even intervals from one heartbeat to the next	

Intervention
Increased variability

Observe the FHR tracing carefully for any sign of fetal distress, including decreasing variability and late decelerations. Consider using the internal mode (spiral electrode) of monitoring if the pattern is observed during external monitoring, especially if it is thought to be a precursor of decreased variability.

Decreased variability

Intervention is dependent on the cause. Intervention is not warranted if decreased variability is associated with fetal sleep cycles or if it is temporarily associated with central nervous system depressants. Application of the spiral electrode should be considered if the pattern is observed using external monitoring. If a CNS-depressant drug has been given and delivery appears imminent, Narcan may be administered to the mother before delivery and is routinely administered to the neonate after delivery. If hypoxia is suspected, turning the patient on her side and administering oxygen may be of some value. In addition, hydration and elimination of uterine hyperstimulation may enhance fetal oxygenation and uteroplacental blood flow.

Tachycardia

Description

Fetal tachycardia is defined as a baseline heart rate above 160 bpm or more than 30 bpm from the normal baseline for a duration of 10 minutes or more (Figure 5-5). Tachycardia has been described as moderate or marked. Moderate tachycardia is defined as a rate between 161 and 180 bpm. This rate has been associated with mild hypoxia or a fetus who is becoming progressively more hypoxic. Marked tachycardia is defined by a FHR greater than 180 bpm. When accompanied by periodic FHR changes and/or minimal or absent variability, a FHR greater than 180 bpm is considered to be a nonreassuring sign.

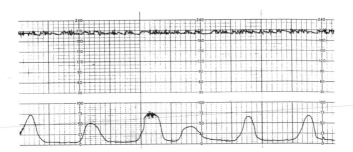

Figure 5-5
Fetal tachycardia.

Causes

1. Fetal hypoxia	1. Fetus attempts to compensate for reduced blood flow by increase of sympathetic stimulation or release of epinephrine from adrenal medulla, or both
2. Maternal fever	2. Accelerates metabolism of fetal myocardium; increases sympathetic cardioacceleration activity up to 2 hours before the mother is febrile
3. Parasympatholytic drugs (e.g., atropine, scopolamine, hydroxyzine [Vistaril, Atarax], phenothiazines)	3. Block the parasympathetic division of the autonomic nervous system
4. Betasympathomimetic drugs (e.g., terbutaline and ritodrine)	4. These tocolytic drugs, given to control labor, have a cardiac stimulant effect similar to that of epinephrine
5. Ilicit drugs (e.g., cocaine and methamphetamines)	5. Epinephrine/norepinephrine response that causes increased maternal and fetal heart rate.
6. Amnionitis	6. Increased heart rate can be the first sign of developing intrauterine infection (as with prolonged rupture of membranes)
7. Maternal hyperthyroidism	7. Long-acting thyroid stimulating hormones (LATS) probably cross the placenta and increase the fetal heart rate, if maternal hyperthyroidism is controlled
8. Fetal anemia	8. FHR increases in an effort to increase cardiac output and tissue perfusion
9. Fetal heart failure	9. The fetal heart attempts to compensate for failure by concurrently increasing rate and cardiac output; can occur as a result of tachyarrhythmia

Variations in Variability Appearance and Cause	Clinical Significance/Intervention
10. Fetal cardiac dysrhythmias*	10. Tachyarrhythmias and variations of normal sinus rhythm may occur (e.g., paroxysmal atrial tachycardia [PAT], atrial flutter, and premature ventricular contractions [PVCs]); congenital cardiac anomaly may be present; FHR in excess of 240 bpm cannot be followed by monitor because this exceeds FHR range parameters

Clinical Significance

Three types of fetal tachycardia are sinus tachycardia, atrial flutter/fibrillation, and supraventricular tachycardia. Sinus tachycardia, with a rate above 160 bpm, may be the result of a drug effect or a response to maternal infection such as amnionitis. It is not necessarily a sign of fetal hypoxia unless it is associated with repetitive late decelerations and/or lack of variability. Atrial flutter/fibrillation, with an atrial rate between 300 and 450 bpm, is rarely diagnosed in the antepartum period and is associated with a high mortality rate.

Supraventricular tachycardia (SVT), with a heart rate in excess of 200 bpm, is the most frequently occurring form of fetal tachyarrhythmia. Short periods of SVT are of no clinical significance. However, longer periods of SVT have been associated with high cardiac output failure, nonimmune hydrops fetalis, ascites, polyhydramnios, and fetal death.

Tachycardia can be a nonreassuring sign when associated with late decelerations or absence of variability. In terms of immediate neonatal outcome, persistent tachycardia with average baseline variability or in the absence of periodic changes (e.g., decelerations) does not appear serious. This is particularly true when tachycardia is associated with maternal fever.

* *Fetal cardiac dysrhythmias* may be confused with electrical noise or maternal ECG artifact on the fetal monitor since they are characterized by large vertical excursions on the FHR scale. They can, however, be diagnosed through the use of spiral electrode, real-time ultrasound, and turning off the logic switch and checking EFM for malfunction.

Intervention

Intervention for tachycardia is dependent on etiological factors. Maternal fever can be reduced with antipyretics, hydration, and cooling measures. If maternal oxygenation is an issue, oxygen at 8 to 10 L/min at 100% via snug face mask may improve or enhance fetal oxygenation and uteroplacental blood flow. When the diagnosis of SVT is made, in utero therapy of the premature fetus or delivery of the mature fetus must be initiated. In utero treatment can consist of maternal administration of a single drug or combinations of digoxin, calcium channel blockers (nifedipine), beta-blockers (propranolol [Inderal]), and antiarrhythmic agents such as procainamide and quinidine, which cross placental barriers and treat the fetus.

Bradycardia

Description

Fetal bradycardia (Figure 5-6) is defined as a baseline heart rate below 120 bpm (or if fetus is >40 weeks gestation, less than 110 bpm) or less than 30 bpm from the normal baseline for a duration of 10 minutes or more (standard definition found in many sources including AWHONN (NAACOG), 1992). However, in most institutions, it is standard practice that clinical intervention begins within 2 to 3 minutes of the beginning of a bradycardic episode of a FHR <110 bpm. During labor, heart rates between 100 and 119 bpm are thought to be a benign change caused by a vagal response to head compression. When associated with periodic FHR changes, heart

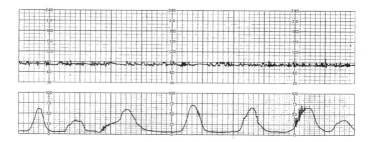

Figure 5-6
Fetal bradycardia.

rates below 100 bpm are the result of progressive fetal acidosis and are considered to be nonreassuring.

Causes

1. Late (profound) fetal hypoxia

2. Beta-adrenergic blocking drugs (e.g.,propran- olol)

3. Anesthetics (epidural, spinal, and pudendal)

4. Maternal hypotension

5. Prolonged umbilical cord compression

6. Fetal cardiac dysrhythmias

7. Hypothermia

8. Maternal systemic lupus erythematosus

9. Cytomegalovirus (CMV)

10. Prolonged maternal hypoglycemia

1. Myocardial activity becomes depressed and lowers heart rate

2. Epinephrine receptor sites in the myocardium are blocked by these drugs, permitting unopposed vagal tone and a decreased heart rate

3. Bradycardia may develop indirectly because of a reflex mechanism or because of maternal hypotension produced by maternal supine position, insufficient preanesthesia hydration, or the response to the anesthetic agent

4. Maternal supine position causes uterine compression of the vena cava, which results in hypotension syndrome (a decrease in cardiac output and blood pressure with a subsequent decrease in FHR)

5. Cord compression triggers sensitization of fetal baroceptors, resulting in vagal stimulation and decreased heart rate

6. FHR can be low (70 to 90 bpm) with bradyarrhythmias (complete heart block)

7. Maternal (and therefore fetal) hypothermia reduces myocardial metabolism, decreases oxygen requirements, and decreases heart rate

8. Complete atrioventricular dissociation associated with connective tissue disease produces persistent bradycardia

9. Structural cardiac defects may occur with CMV infection, resulting in congenital heart block expressed as fetal bradycardia

10. Maternal and subsequently fetal hypoglycemia can potentiate hypoxemia

	with a depression of myocardial activity and decreased heart rate
11. Congenital heart block	11. Congenital heart block of first, second, or third degree can result in bradycardia. First-degree block does not require treatment in the fetus and has not yet been reported in the literature. In second-degree block not all the impulses from the sinoatrial node in the atria are conducted to the ventricles. Mobitz type I block is evidenced by a progressive lengthening of the PR interval and is rarely of any significance. Mobitz type II block occurs infrequently but is more serious and often a precursor to third-degree heart block.

Clinical Significance

Bradycardia resulting from hypoxia is a nonreassuring sign when associated with loss of variability and late decelerations. Long-term bradycardia that is unresponsive to intervention indicates advanced fetal distress and may be a preterminal event. Bradycardia with average FHR variability and absence of late decelerations is not a sign of fetal distress and should be considered benign. Intervention is also not warranted in fetuses with heart block diagnosed in the antepartum period.

Although paracervical blocks are now rarely performed, the resultant bradycardia is usually transitory with recovery occurring in utero. The 5-minute Apgar is usually above 7 if the FHR pattern was reassuring before the onset of the bradycardia and if delivery does not occur during the paracervical block bradycardia. Poor fetal outcome has occurred with delivery during the resulting bradycardia caused by fetal hypoxia and acidosis. Neonatal resuscitation and stabilization is indicated until the paracervical pharmacological agent has been metabolized.

Intervention

Intervention for bradycardia is dependent on etiological factors. Clinical judgment and resulting intervention are based on a variety of factors, including stage of labor, presentation and station of fetus, and indications of fetal stress. Maternal positioning (lateral), hydration, correction of maternal hypotension, maternal oxygenation at 8 to 10 L/min at 100% by snug face mask, and elimination of uterine hyperstimulation are indicated to improve fetal oxygenation and uteroplacental blood flow. In addition, scalp stimulation can be performed in an effort to produce FHR acceleration in order to establish whether the fetus has the ability to mobilize oxygen and physiologically compensate for stress. Infants delivered with congenital heart block may require a pacemaker.

Unusual Patterns
Sinusoidal Pattern

A sinusoidal fetal heart rate pattern (Figure 5-7) is characterized by the following features:
1. A heart rate between 120 and 160 bpm
2. Regular oscillations with an amplitude of 5 to 15 bpm
3. Frequency of 2 to 5 cycles per minute of long-term variability
4. Minimal to absent short-term variability
5. Rhythmic oscillation of a sine wave above and below a baseline
6. Absence of FHR accelerations in response to fetal movement

This pattern has been known to occur in the presence of fetal hypoxia, often as a result of Rh isoimmunization, fetal anemia, and chronic fetal bleeds. In these cases it has been associated with an increase in fetal morbidity and mortality, and survival may depend on extrauterine support and in a neonatal intensive care unit.

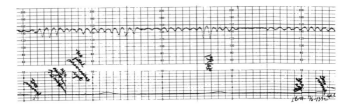

Figure 5-7
Sinusoidal FHR.
(Courtesy Roger K. Freeman, M.D., Long Beach, Calif.)

The pattern has also been reported after the administration of analgesics, such as alphaprodine (Nisentil), meperidine (Demerol), and butorphanol tartrate (Stadol), and in association with amnionitis. The sinusoidal pattern following the administration of these drugs is usually a temporary phenomenon not associated with an adverse fetal outcome and the pattern may be corrected after a dose of Narcan.

Expeditious delivery may be indicated if there is a persistent, uncorrectable sinusoidal pattern and other signs of fetal distress are present. If the pattern is inconsistent and apparently transitory after intravenous narcotics, fetal compromise is not expected.

Fetal Cardiac Dysrhythmias

Fetal cardiac dysrhythmias occur in many pregnancies. Tachycardia and bradycardia have been previously discussed in this chapter. Other dysrhythmias include:

1. Premature atrial contractions (PACs) and premature ventricular contractions (PVCs)

1. These are represented on the tracing as vertical excursions above or below the FHR baseline. PACs and PVCs usually have no clinical significance and do not require intervention.

2. Transient fetal cardiac asystole

2. Transient fetal cardiac asystole may be evidenced by a rapid downward deflection of the FHR followed quickly by a rapid upward excursion back to the previous FHR baseline. This has been reported during the nadir of severe variable decelerations. Management should include position change, vaginal examination to rule out cord prolapse or rapid fetal descent, and elevation of the presenting part as indicated.

It is important to distinguish fetal dysrhythmias from electrical noise or maternal ECG artifact, since they can all be evidenced by the same pattern. To adequately discriminate fetal dysrhythmias from noise and artifact, diagnoses can be achieved by spiral electrode, real-time ultrasound, and turning off the logic switch and checking EFM for malfunction.

Summary of Baseline Changes

	Tachycardia
Definition	Sustained FHR above 160 bpm for more than 10 minutes
Etiology	Early fetal hypoxia, drugs, maternal fever, amnionitis, fetal anemia, fetal heart failure, and/or cardiac arrhythmias
Clinical significance	Usually benign when associated with maternal fever
	Nonreassuring when associated with late decelerations, loss of variability, or severe variable decelerations
Nursing intervention	Dependent on etiological factors; reduce maternal fever with hydration, antipyretics, and cooling measures; lateral position change and oxygen at 8 to 10 L/min by snug face mask may be of some value
	For supraventricular tachycardia, in utero treatment can consist of maternal administration of a single drug or combinations of digoxin, calcium channel blockers (nifedipine), beta-blockers (propranolol [Inderal]), and antiarrhythmic agents such as procainamide and quinidine, which cross placental barriers and treat the fetus

Bradycardia	Minimal to Absent Variability
Sustained FHR below 120 bpm for more than 10 minutes	*Short term:* changes in FHR from one beat to the next
	Long term: rhythmic fluctuations in the baseline about 3 to 5 cycles per minute
Late (profound) fetal hypoxia, drugs, maternal hypotension, prolapsed cord, or congenital heart block	*Decreased variability:* prematurity, drugs, hypoxia, fetal sleep, congenital abnormalities, fetal cardiac arrhythmias, CNS depression
Bradycardia without periodic deceleration and with average FHR variability is not a sign of fetal hypoxia	Benign when associated with periodic fetal sleep; return of variability usually occurs when drugs are excreted or metabolized
Nonreassuring when associated with late decelerations or loss of variability; indicates profound fetal distress	Ominous when associated with late decelerations
Dependent on etiological factors; lateral position change and oxygen at 8 to 10 L/min by snug face mask may be of some value; eliminate uterine hyperstimulation to improve fetal oxygenation and uteroplacental blood flow; scalp stimulation can be performed in an effort to produce FHR acceleration to establish whether the fetus has the ability to mobilize oxygen and physiologically compensate for stress. Intervention is not warranted in fetus with heart block diagnosed by ECG in the antepartum period	Dependent on etiological factors; fetal blood sampling for pH may provide additional clinical information; intervention is not warranted if associated with fetal sleep cycle or temporarily associated with central nervous system depressants

Periodic and Nonperiodic Changes

6

Periodic changes in FHR are transient accelerations or decelerations from the baseline, after which the FHR returns to baseline. These changes usually occur in response to uterine contractions and may begin as compensatory mechanisms or precursors to hypoxia. They are classified as uniform accelerations and decelerations.

Nonperiodic changes are accelerations or decelerations that occur without any specific relationship to uterine activity. They can include spontaneous accelerations and variable decelerations between contractions and prolonged decelerations.

All FHR changes, whether periodic or nonperiodic, should be systematically evaluated within the parameters of the "company they keep" (Chez, 1992). These parameters include FHR baseline and variability before, during, and after the change; presence of combined changes (e.g., lates and variables); change related to uterine activity or resting tone (e.g., hyperstimulation and increased resting tone); and general information that is available about maternal and fetal condition. By doing this complete assessment, the clinician remains aware of changes that suggest levels of hypoxia (mild to worsening), as well as the presence or absence of compensatory mechanisms that give an indication of the level of oxygen reserve in fetal tissue. Timely and appropriate interventions then follow the evaluation of the FHR pattern and determination of fetal stress tolerance.

Accelerations

Description

Accelerations of FHR from the baseline are most often associated with fetal movement (spontaneous) and uterine contractions (periodic). They can also occur before or after variable decelerations.

82

Accelerations are transitory increases above the baseline and may resemble the shape of uterine contractions. The onset is variable, often preceding or occurring simultaneously with uterine contractions or fetal movement. The recovery is variable and the amplitude is usually 15 or more bpm from the baseline (Figure 6-1).

Characteristics

	Spontaneous*	Uniform/Periodic
SHAPE	Spike-like or transitory increase in baseline	Resembles shape of uterine contraction
ONSET	Variable, can occur any-time	Before or after peak of uterine contraction
RECOVERY	Variable	Return to baseline can occur after or at the same time as the uterine pressure returns to its resting tone
ACCELERATION	Usually 15 bpm above baseline	Variable; usually 10 to 15 bpm above baseline
BASELINE	Associated with average baseline variability	Sometimes associated with decreasing or smooth baseline variability
OCCURRENCE	Variable; not associated with uterine contraction or periodic decelerations; in response to fetal stimulation	Repetitious; tends to occur with each contraction; has occurred in some cases before the onset of late decelerations

*See discussion of spontaneous (nonperiodic) accelerations on page 102.

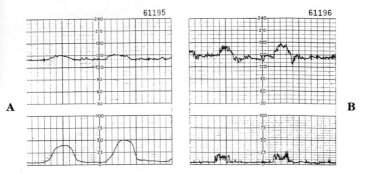

Figure 6-1
A, Acceleration of FHR with uterine contractions. **B,** Acceleration of FHR with fetal movement.

Etiology

Stimulation of the sympathetic division of the autonomic nervous system can accelerate the FHR. Acceleration can result from the following:

1. Spontaneous fetal movement
2. Vaginal examination
3. Electrode application
4. Breech presentation
5. Occiput posterior presentation
6. Uterine contractions
7. Fundal pressure
8. Abdominal palpation

Uniform accelerations of >15 bpm above baseline for >15 seconds in response to contractions are caused by an increase in beta-adrenergic sympathetic stimulation of the autonomic nervous system. These accelerations indicate an intact CNS pathway.

Clinical Significance

Spontaneous acceleration of FHR of ≥15 bpm for ≥15 seconds in response to fetal movement and uterine contractions is an indication of fetal central nervous system (CNS) alertness and well-being and is reassuring. Fetal movement can be observed on the uterine activity panel as spikes or momentary increases in uterine pressure on the lower section of the monitor strip.

Repetitive uniform accelerations occurring in connection with uterine contractions indicate an initial response to mild hypoxia.

This is secondary to baroreceptor-induced transient increase in FHR that occurs as a result of fetal hypotension produced when a uterine contraction compresses the umbilical vein without compressing the umbilical artery. This compensatory mechanism reflects a healthy fetus with an appropriate cardiovascular response to stress.

As labor progresses, uniform accelerations are seen as precursors to increased cord compression and, later, variable decelerations. This combination of changes (acceleration to variable deceleration) has been frequently associated with breech presentation because of increased cord vulnerability during uterine contractions (Cabaniss, 1993).

Intervention

Acceleration of FHR is considered a benign pattern, and no intervention is required. If partial cord compression is suspected, maternal repositioning can be done. However, it would be wise to observe uniform accelerations just in case they are followed by a small deceleration they can evolve into a pattern of variable or late decelerations as labor progresses.

Early Decelerations

Description

Early decelerations, or head compression decelerations, are those that begin early in the contracting phase with the onset before the peak of the uterine contraction and the recovery occurring at the same time the uterine contraction returns to the baseline. The timing is synchronous with that of the contraction. Generally this pattern occurs with advanced dilatation (>7 cm).

Physiology

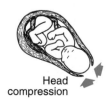

Head
compression

Pressure on the fetal skull
↓
Alters cerebral blood flow
↓
Stimulates central vagus nerve
↓
Produces decrease in heart rate with
↓
Recovery occurring as pressure
  is relieved

Characteristics (Figure 6-2)

SHAPE	Uniform shape; a "mirror image" of the contraction phase
ONSET	Early in the contraction phase; before the peak of the contraction; nadir, or low point, of the deceleration occurs at the peak of the contraction
RECOVERY	Return to baseline occurs by the end of the contraction as uterine pressure returns to its resting tone
DECELERATION	Rarely decelerates below 110 bpm, or 20 to 30 bpm below baseline; amplitude of deceleration is usually proportional to amplitude of contraction
BASELINE	Usually associated with average baseline variability
OCCURRENCE	Repetitious; occurs with each contraction; usually observed between 4 and 7 cm dilatation and, in second stage, as fetal head descends through pelvis

Etiology

This pattern is a result of direct vagal stimulation of the temporal baroreceptors as a result of descent and increased pressure on the head as it passes through the pelvic outlet and vaginal canal. Head compression decelerations can result from the following:

1. Uterine contractions
2. Vaginal examinations
3. Fundal pressure
4. Placement of internal scalp electrode

Clinical Significance

Early or head compression deceleration has no pathological significance. It is usually a benign pattern not associated with fetal hypoxia or acidosis. It is not usually associated with other heart rate changes, such as tachycardia.

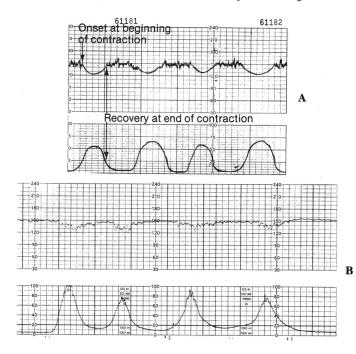

Figure 6-2
A, Early deceleration (illustration with key points identified).
B, Early deceleration (actual tracing).

Intervention

Early deceleration is a benign pattern and no intervention is required. The importance of identifying early decelerations is to be able to distinguish them from late and variable decelerations.

Late Decelerations
Description

Late decelerations are those that begin late in the contracting phase with the onset at or after the peak of the uterine contraction and the recovery occurring after the return of the contraction to the baseline. They are generally proportional to uterine contractions and thus are readily observed with stronger contractions and not as evident with weaker contractions.

Physiology

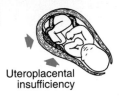

Uteroplacental
insufficiency

Uterine hyperactivity
  or maternal hypo-
  tension

True placental
dysfunction

↓

Decreases intervillous
  space blood flow
  during uterine
  contractions

↓

Decreases maternal/fetal oxygen transfer

↓   ↓

Produces fetal
  hypoxia and myo-
  cardial depression

↓

Activates vagal
  response

Anaerobic
metabolism

↓   ↓

Produces cardio-
  deceleration ←————— Lactic acidosis

Characteristics (Figure 6-3)

SHAPE   Uniform shape; a "mirror image" of the
                 contraction phase, deep or shallow depending
                 upon the degree of hypoxia

ONSET   Late in the contraction phase at or after the peak
                 of the contraction; nadir, or low point, of the
                 deceleration occurs well after the peak of the
                 contraction

RECOVERY   Return to the baseline occurs after the end of the
                 contraction (usually more than 20 seconds
                 after uterine pressure returns to its resting
                 tone)

DECELERATION   Rarely decelerates below 100 bpm; amplitude of
                 deceleration is usually proportional to ampli-

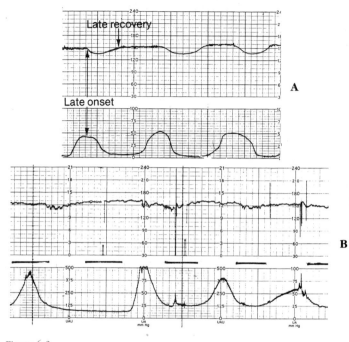

Figure 6-3

A, Late deceleration (illustration with key points identified). **B,** Late deceleration (actual tracing).

tude of contraction; *persistent, uncorrected decelerations of any magnitude are nonreassuring,* and the most depressed fetuses may have only shallow late decelerations (e.g., 3 to 5 bpm)

BASELINE   Often associated with loss of variability and a rising baseline or tachycardia; variability may be increased or decreased during the nadir of the deceleration

OCCURRENCE   Repetitious; occurs with each contraction; can be observed at any time during labor when there is uteroplacental insufficiency

Etiology

Uteroplacental insufficiency can result from the following:

Cause	Effect
1. Hyperstimulation of the uterus from oxytocin augmentation or induction	1. Hyperstimulation enhances vasoconstriction, reduces cardiac output, and decreases intervillous space blood flow
2. Maternal spine hypotension	2. Compression of the inferior vena cava reduces venous return and maternal cardiac output
3. Pregnancy-induced hypertension	3. Vasospasm occurring in uterine vessels decreases intervillous space blood flow and produces fetal hypoxia
4. Chronic hypertension	4. Hypertensive vascular disease constricts blood vessels and reduces intervillous blood flow, thus producing fetal hypoxia
5. Postmaturity	5. Fetus "outgrows" placenta; insufficient function of the placenta reduces supply of oxygen and nutrients to the fetus
6. Amnionitis	6. Maternal infection reduces the efficiency of the uteroplacental unit; related fetal tachycardia increases the metabolic rate, rapidly depleting placental oxygen reserves; amnionitis often causes uterine hyperactivity, which decreases intervillous space blood flow and leads to fetal hypoxia
7. Small-for-gestational-age (SGA)	7. Intrauterine growth retardation (IUGR) with reduced fetal placental reserve

Cause	Effect
8. Maternal diabetes	8. Maternal vascular involvement and sclerotic arterial changes reduce uteroplacental perfusion
9. Placenta previa	9. Placental attachment to the lower uterine segment (covering internal cervical os) may cause early separation and increase chance of hemorrhage
10. Abruptio placentae/maternal shock	10. Premature separation of placenta decreases functioning placental area and related uterine hyperactivity
11. Regional anesthetics (spinal, epidural)	11. May cause maternal hypotension, reducing blood flow to uteroplacental unit
12. Maternal cardiac disease	12. Conditions that affect pumping of blood reduce blood flow to uteroplacental unit; cyanotic conditions reduce oxygen content of blood flowing to placenta
13. Maternal anemia	13. Reduction of RBCs or hemoglobin decreases the amount of oxygen to fetoplacental unit
14. Rh isoimmunization	14. Fetal anemia decreases the amount of available oxygen and the hypoxic stress occurring with a uterine contraction can precipitate metabolic acidosis
15. Other conditions; collagen vascular disease, renal disease, and advanced maternal age	15. Conditions compromise placental exchange because of sclerotic arterial and venous changes

Clinical Significance

Late decelerations of any magnitude should be considered a nonreassuring sign when they are persistent and uncorrectable, especially
when associated with tachycardia and/or minimal or absent variability. As myocardial depression increases, the depth of the late deceleration decreases, becoming more subtle or shallow in appearance. In contrast, a single late deceleration in an otherwise
reassuring pattern is not clinically significant.

Persistent and uncorrectable late decelerations reflect repetitive
hypoxic stress and if associated with minimal or absent variability
become a sign of increasing metabolic acidosis.

Intervention

Procedure*	Rationale
1. Change maternal position to lateral	1. Decreases pressure on the inferior vena cava and corrects supine hypotension

2. Correct maternal hypotension
   a. Lower head
	2.
	   a. Increases venous return and promotes cardiac output

b. Increase rate of maintenance IV infusion	b. Increases maternal circulating volume and cardiac output; this can facilitate excretion of oxytocin
c. Administer vasopressors (e.g., ephedrine sulfate)	c. Increases blood pressure by increasing arteriolar constriction and cardiac stimulation
3. Discontinue oxytocin if infusing	3. Decreases uterine activity
4. Administer oxygen 8 to 10 L/min at 100% by snug face mask	4. Increases maternal oxygen saturation of hemoglobin
5. Fetal scalp or acoustic stimulation	5. May be useful to elicit an acceleration of FHR that would not be indicative of fetal acidosis

* Consider placement of internal electrode as appropriate for better assessment of
potential problems.

6. Termination of labor is considered by the physician if the pattern cannot be corrected, particularly if variability is decreasing and an acceleration of FHR cannot be elicited

6. Continuation of labor can only further compromise the fetus by increasing hypoxia and acidosis

Variable Decelerations

Description

Variable decelerations are those that occur with any interruption in umbilical blood flow during the uterine contracting phase but are often concurrent with uterine contractions. The decelerations vary in intensity and duration (usually <2 minutes) and frequently decelerate below the average FHR range. Variable deceleration patterns are the most frequently observed FHR pattern in labor.

Physiology

Umbilical cord compression

Transitory umbilical cord compression
↓
Collapses umbilical vein → Producing fetal hypovolemia
↓   ↓
Occludes umbilical ← Transient cardio-acceleration
artery/vein
↓
Produces hemodynamic changes (hypotension from fetal outflow of blood without return from placenta)
↓
Activates baroceptors and chemoceptors
↓
Stimulates vagus nerve
↓
Produces cardiodeceleration ←
↓
(reflective of baroceptor response to final hypertension with total occlusion)
↓
if prolonged ⟶ produces hypoxia

Characteristics

SHAPE	Variable; does not reflect the shape of any associated uterine contraction; characterized by a sudden drop in heart rate in a $\vee$ or $\vee$ shape (u, v, or w shape)
ONSET	Variable times in the contraction phase; often preceded and followed by transitory acceleration (shouldering) signifying compensation for umbilical vein occlusion
RECOVERY	Return to baseline occurs rapidly, sometimes with transitory acceleration (shouldering);$\vee$, or $\vee$overshoot
DECELERATION	Often decelerates below 100 bpm
BASELINE	May be associated with average baseline variability or decreased variability with significant hypoxia
OCCURRENCE	Not necessarily repetitive; frequently observed late in labor; may be associated with pushing in the second stage of labor

Variations (Figures 6-4 to 6-6)

Mild: decelerates to any level less than 30 seconds with abrupt return to baseline

Moderate: decelerates no less than 80 bpm, any duration with abrupt return to baseline

Severe: decelerates below 60 bpm or 60 bpm below baseline for greater than 60 seconds with slow return to baseline (baseline rate may increase while baseline variability decreases)

Etiology

Interruption in umbilical blood flow can result from the following:
1. Maternal position; cord between fetus and maternal pelvis
2. Cord around fetal neck, leg, arm, or other body part
3. Short cord
4. Knot in cord
5. Prolapsed cord

Clinical Significance

Variable decelerations occur in about 50% of all labors and are usually transient and correctable phenomena. They vary in duration,

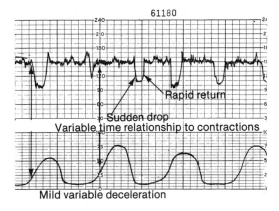

Figure 6-4
Mild variable decelerations (illustration with key points
identified).

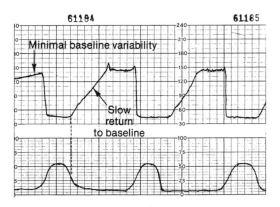

Figure 6-5
Severe variable decelerations (illustration with key points
identified).

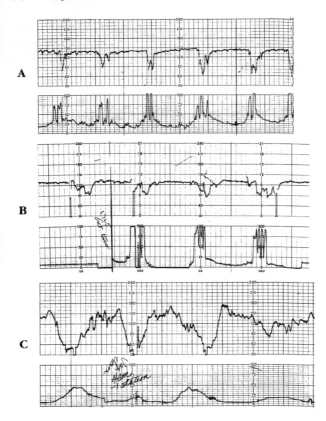

Figure 6-6
A, Mild variable deceleration. **B,** Moderate variable
deceleration. **C,** Severe variable decelerations (all are actual
tracings).

depth (nadir), and timing relative to uterine contraction and any
other type of interruption in umbilical blood flow.

Reassuring variable decelerations (Freeman, Garite, and Nageotte,
1991):

1. Last no more than 30 to 45 seconds
2. Have a rapid return to baseline (no evidence of a late compo-
   nent/slow return)
3. Baseline rate is not increasing
4. Variability is not decreasing

Transitory umbilical cord compression is associated with respiratory acidosis, which is rapidly corrected when cord compression is relieved.

Shouldering, or a transitory acceleration of the FHR preceding and following the deceleration, indicates the interaction of the sympathetic and parasympathetic nervous systems and a baroreceptor response to hypotension produced by a transient "vein-only" phase of umbilical cord compression (Cabaniss, 1993). Shouldering is generally associated with normal or increased variability, and is evaluated as an appropriate compensatory response to the stress of umbilical cord compression.

An overshoot, a smooth transitory acceleration of FHR upon return to baseline, indicates the presence of significant hypoxic stress and is a nonreassuring sign. Overshoots generally follow moderate and severe variable decelerations, have absent short-term variability, and usually last >20 to 30 seconds.

Severe variable decelerations just before delivery are usually well tolerated if the total time is short from the onset of the decelerations to the time of delivery, and if the neonate is able to eliminate excess respiratory carbon dioxide.

A progressively slower return to baseline with repetitive severe variable decelerations indicates a gradual increase in hypoxia. Severe uncorrectable variable decelerations, particularly with loss of short-term variability and a rise in baseline rate, are associated with fetal acidosis, hypoxia, and a neurologically depressed newborn.

Intervention

Procedure*	Rationale
1. Change maternal position from side to side, Trendelenburg, or knee-chest	1. May relieve cord compression
2. When decelerations are severe:	2. Pattern may be a warning or nonreassuring sign of fetal distress
a. Discontinue oxytocin if infusing	a. Decreases uterine activity, which can contribute to cord compression

*Consider placement of internal electrode as appropriate for better assessment of potential problems.

b. Administer oxygen 8 to 10 L/min at 100% by snug face mask (maximum increase in fetal SaO$_2$ occurs *only* after approximately 9 minutes of 100% O$_2$ administration to mother [McNamara, Johnson, and Lilford, 1993])

b. Increases maternal oxygen saturation of hemoglobin in an attempt to raise fetal PO$_2$ when cord is decompressed

c. Vaginal or speculum examination, or both

c. Checks for prolapsed umbilical cord or imminent delivery

d. Amnioinfusion may be of some value

d. Instillation of normal saline through the intrauterine catheter may relieve cord compression (see Chapter 7)

e. Termination of labor is considered by the physician if the severe variable deceleration pattern cannot be corrected. (If the pattern is corrected enough to be reassuring, the labor can be allowed to continue)

e. Continuation of severe variable decelerations can only further compromise the fetus by increasing hypoxia and acidosis

Summary of Periodic Changes: Decelerations (Figure 6-7)

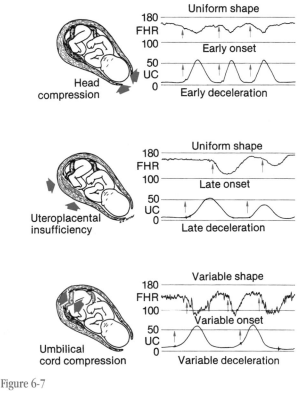

Figure 6-7
Summary of periodic changes.

	Early
Etiology	Head compression/vagal response
Onset	Early; before peak of uterine contraction (UC)
Recovery	By end of contraction as uterine pressure returns to resting tone
Deceleration	Rarely decelerates below 110 bpm
Clinical significance	Compensatory
Nursing intervention	Observe for changes of pattern

Late	Variable
Uteroplacental insufficiency	Any interruption in umbilical blood flow
Late; at or after peak of UC, with nadir, or low point, well after peak of UC	Variable; anytime between or during contractions
After end of UC, well after pressure has returned to resting tone	Variable; may have rapid return, prolonged return, shouldering over baseline (compensatory) or overshoot (nonreassuring)
Can decelerate any amount but is usually within normal FHR range of 120 to 160 bpm	Often decelerates below normal FHR range
Nonreassuring	May be transient; may progress to nonreassuring
Change maternal position	Change maternal position
Correct maternal hypotension; elevate legs; increase rate of maintenance IV infusion	Continue with the following only for severe variable decelerations:
Discontinue oxytocin if infusing	Discontinue oxytocin if infusing
Administer oxygen 8 to 10 L/min at 100% by snug face mask	Administer oxygen 8 to 10 L/min at 100% by snug face mask
Fetal scalp or acoustic stimulation, pH, or termination of labor may be indicated	Vaginal or speculum examination, or both; amnioinfusion; termination of labor may be indicated if severe variable decelerations are not correctable

Nonperiodic Changes
Description

Nonperiodic changes include spontaneous accelerations, variable decelerations as the umbilical cord is compressed between contractions (e.g., nuchal or shoulder cord, or with oligohydramnios), and prolonged variable decelerations.

Spontaneous Accelerations
Description

Spontaneous accelerations of FHR from the baseline are most often associated with fetal movement and may resemble a spike-like or transitory increase above baseline as a result of sympathetic nervous system stimulation. The onset, frequency, duration, and amplitude are variable.

Characteristics

SHAPE	Spike-like, or transitory increase above baseline
ONSET	Variable, can occur anytime
RECOVERY	Variable
ACCELERATION	Usually 15 bpm above baseline
BASELINE	Associated with average baseline variability
OCCURRENCE	Variable; not associated with uterine contraction or periodic decelerations; in response to fetal stimulation

Etiology

Spontaneous accelerations as a result of stimulation of the sympathetic division of the autonomic nervous system can result from the following:
1. Spontaneous fetal movement
2. Vaginal examination/electrode application
3. Fundal pressure/abdominal palpation

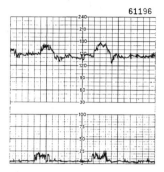

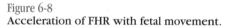

Figure 6-8
Acceleration of FHR with fetal movement.

Clinical Significance

Spontaneous accelerations of FHR >15 bpm for ≥15 seconds are an indication of central nervous system alertness and are considered reassuring (Figure 6-8). Conversely, the absence of spontaneous accelerations without just cause (e.g., during the normal 30 to 40 minutes of an average fetal sleep cycle), and/or in the presence of decreased or absent variability and/or late decelerations is nonreassuring.

Intervention

In the absence of spontaneous accelerations, further evaluation of ability of FHR to accelerate (via scalp or acoustic stimulation) is warranted and intervention may be required to attempt to improve fetal oxygenation.

Prolonged Decelerations

Description

Generally a prolonged deceleration is an isolated event. It is most frequently associated with occult or frank cord prolapse and progressive severe variable decelerations. It is characterized by a prolonged deceleration of 60 to 90 seconds or more below the average FHR range.

Characteristics (Figure 6-9)

SHAPE	Variable in shape; does not reflect the shape of any associated uterine contraction
ONSET	Variable times in the contracting phase
RECOVERY	May last 90 seconds or more, with a loss of variability and rebound tachycardia; occasionally a period of late decelerations follows; some fetuses do not recover and the result is fetal death
DECELERATION	Deceleration is almost always below the normal FHR range
BASELINE	Often associated with a loss of variability and postdeceleration tachycardia
OCCURRENCE	Usually isolated events but may be seen late in the course of repetitive, severe variable decelerations or during a prolonged series of late decelerations and just before fetal death

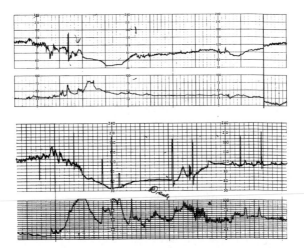

Figure 6-9
Prolonged decelerations.

Etiology

1. Cord compression

1. A sudden occult or frank prolapse of umbilical cord

2. Maternal hypotension (supine or related to epidural or spinal anesthesia)

2. Profound uteroplacental insufficiency may result from hypotension, causing a prolonged deceleration

3. Paracervical anesthesia

3. Possibly related to fetal uptake of anesthetic agent, local hypotension from uterine artery spasms, or uterine hypertonus

4. Tetanic uterine contractions (oxytocin stimulation, abruptio placentae, or related to a problem with administration of epidural anesthesia)

4. Hypertonic contractions result in uteroplacental insufficiency; inadvertent intravenous injection of anesthetic with an epidural block can result in a tetanic contraction and prolonged deceleration; breast hyperstimulation; *cocaine ingestion* with vasospasm, hypertonus, and abruptio placentae

5. Maternal hypoxia

5. Maternal seizure activity or respiratory depression (from narcotic overdose, magnesium sulfate toxicity, or high spinal anesthetic)

6. Procedures and physiological mechanisms: spiral electrode application; pelvic examination; sustained maternal Valsalva; rapid fetal descent through the birth canal

6. Fetal head compression/ stimulation can produce a strong vagal response, cardiodeceleration, and a prolonged deceleration

Clinical Significance

Prolonged deceleration(s) associated with fetal head compression (spiral electrode application, pelvic examination, sustained maternal Valsalva, rapid fetal descent) usually lasts for only 1 to 2 minutes and recovers with predeceleration variability and baseline. Decelerations caused by maternal hypotension, tetanic contractions, and maternal hypoxia generally occur with some loss of variability and tachycardia or recurrent late decelerations. If a subsequent prolonged deceleration does not recur, the placenta generally recovers the fetus to its predeceleration state. The prognosis for fetal survival is guarded if the prolonged deceleration occurs after a series of repetitive severe variable decelerations. In this situation prolonged deceleration and/or recurrent late decelerations may result in a terminal bradycardia of 30 to 60 bpm before death.

Intervention

Intervention is based on identifying and alleviating the cause of the prolonged variable deceleration. If the apparent cause is severe uteroplacental insufficiency, umbilical cord compression, or is unidentifiable, then expeditious delivery may be indicated. Measures used to treat fetal distress can be instituted in any case, and these are described in detail under "Intervention for Fetal Distress" in Chapter 7.

Fetal Distress Management

7

The focus of electronic FHR monitoring is to identify the earliest stages of fetal hypoxia and then to intervene in an appropriate and timely manner to prevent fetal asphyxia, which can result from sustained and severe hypoxia. To do this, a knowledge of reassuring, warning, and nonreassuring patterns is essential to the implementation of appropriate interventions. Before reviewing these patterns it must be stated that there is no generally agreed upon precise definition of fetal distress. Hypoxia is considered to be a reduction of oxygen supply to tissue below physiological levels, whereas asphyxia is the end result of profound hypoxia, resulting in anaerobic metabolism and resultant metabolic acidosis.

The diagnosis of birth asphyxia on the basis of fetal pH, Apgar score, and newborn cerebral dysfunction has been described by Gilstrap et al (1989) and should only be applied in the clinical condition defined by the following:

1. Profound umbilical artery metabolic or mixed acidemia (pH < 7.00, base deficit > 20)
2. Five-minute Apgar score of 0 to 3
3. Neonatal neurological sequelae such as seizures, coma, and hypotonia
4. Multiorgan system dysfunction such as the cardiovascular, gastrointestinal, hematologic, renal, and/or pulmonary systems

When comparing fetal stress with distress, variability is the major determinant for assessing the overall level of fetal oxygenation. *Stress* is a change in variability that is correctable by noninvasive intervention (e.g., hydration, change in maternal position, and oxygenation) or by the fetus itself exhibiting its own ability to compensate and centralize oxygen. *Distress* is a change in variability that is not correctable secondary to a breakdown in the fetal compensatory mechanism and results in a progressive loss of variability. The first variability to be lost is in the nadir of

periodic and nonperiodic changes; without intervention it progresses to a decreased, absent, or exaggerated baseline variability
(e.g., saltatory or sinusoidal) and without rescue, will lead to an
adverse outcome.

Research and experience suggest that a previously "normoxic"
fetus can tolerate late or severe decelerations for approximately 30
minutes before showing signs of decompensation. In light of this, it
is crucial for all members of the OB team to agree upon and for-
mulate a plan of action for intervention before the end of any 30-
minute window of nonreassuring FHR tracing that *has not been corrected or shown improvement as a result of interventions* to enhance
uteroplacental blood flow and fetal oxygenation (Parer, 1991).

A number of technologies exist and others are being developed
and tested for the purpose of reducing intrapartum and antepartum
risk to the pregnant woman and her fetus, for example, pulse
oximetry used in labor as a means of measuring fetal oxygen saturation. To date, pulse oximetry use in labor and delivery has been
limited to experimental study and to limited clinical settings in the
United States and internationally (Luttkus, Fengler, Dudenhausen,
1995).

As assessment tools are used and studied, a better understanding
of the fetal response to stress (e.g., uterine contractions) has resulted. Literature and practitioners continue to disagree on the validity, efficacy, and cost effectiveness of surveillance tools and
methods. This is due in part to the lack of agreement about definitions, labels, and parameters that warrant intervention. It is recommended that a chain of command and a plan be developed and
agreed upon by the OB medical, anesthetic, neonatal/pediatric, nursing, and hospital administration staff for interventions of nonreassuring FHR patterns well before intervention is necessary. This plan
should be based on accepted standards of care for the level of institution, resources, and personnel available in each care setting.

Although electronic fetal monitoring was intended to be used as
a reflector of the adequacy of fetal oxygenation and not to reflect
brain function, there are some fetal heart rate patterns that have been
described as usually consistent with existing fetal brain damage.
These include the following:

1. A flat tracing without late decelerations, variable decelerations,
   or prolonged bradycardia has been described with anencephaly
   (VanderMoer et al, Dicker et al, and deHaan et al 1985).

2. A wandering pattern of blunt, slow, irregular undulations with a flat baseline has been reported with anencephaly (Freeman, Garite, and Nageotte, 1991).
3. A sinusoidal EFM pattern has been described in cases of hydrocephalus and severe anemia (Ombelet and VanDer Merwe, 1985; Parer, 1993).
4. A fixed heart rate with late decelerations and terminal bradycardias have been reported to occur in fetuses with severe CNS anomalies (Didolkar and Mutch, 1979).

Literature and practice suggest there is a consensus that an abnormal EFM tracing is a poor predictor of cerebral palsy (CP), even though EFM can identify fetal asphyxia, which can subsequently result in CP. Although this may seem contradictory, in reality (1) EFM can fail to detect severe fetal asphyxia in an undetermined number of cases, (2) perinatal asphyxia is an uncommon cause of CP (possible causes include congenital developmental defects, intrauterine infection, intrauterine exposure to toxins and teratogens, hypothyroidism, and neonatal asphyxia [Hankins, 1991]), and (3) EFM changes that reflect fetal asphyxia and/or acidosis may be the result of a damaged fetal brain and may be a consequence instead of the cause of CP (Niswander, 1991).

In conclusion, the focus of electronic FHR monitoring is to identify patterns that are reassuring and predictive of a positive fetal outcome. To do this, a knowledge of reassuring, warning, and nonreassuring patterns is essential to prompt and appropriate interventions. This chapter describes patterns that are reassuring and considered normal, as well as warning and nonreassuring patterns.

Reassuring Fetal Heart Rate Patterns

A reassuring fetal heart rate pattern (Figure 7-1) is one that is in the average FHR range of 120 to 160 bpm without tachycardia or bradycardia, demonstrates long-term variability (LTV) and the presence of short-term variability (STV) when electronically monitored, is reactive in that there are FHR accelerations with fetal movement, and exhibits an absence of periodic and nonperiodic late and nonreassuring variable decelerations. Presence of variability throughout the baseline is indicative of a fetus with an intact autonomic nervous system and an ability to compensate for periods of stress.

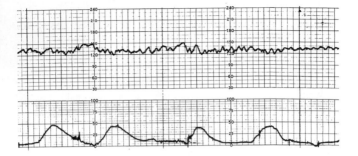

Figure 7-1
Normal FHR and uterine activity pattern.

Description

Baseline rate | 120 to 160 bpm

Short-term variability | More than 6 bpm in amplitude

Long-term variability | 3 to 10 cycles per minute

Periodic changes | Accelerations with fetal movement; early head compression decelerations; reassuring variable decelerations

Normal Uterine Activity Pattern

Frequency | More than 2 minutes between contractions

Duration | Less than 90 seconds

Intensity | Less than 100 mm Hg pressure

Resting tone | Thirty seconds or more between contractions; resting intrauterine pressure less than 20 to 25 mm Hg (can be determined only by intrauterine monitoring)

A reassuring FHR and uterine activity pattern serves to allay the concerns of the patient and staff about the fetal status during labor. This reassuring type of pattern indicates that the fetus is tolerating the process of labor well and does not require any type of intervention. One would expect to have a good fetal outcome with normal Apgar scores and blood gases.

Warning Fetal Heart Rate Patterns

Warning fetal heart rate patterns may be self-limiting, or they may proceed and lead to nonreassuring FHR patterns. If the recording of these patterns is not clear, is of poor quality, or if a more accurate assessment of the pattern is necessary, consider the direct method of monitoring with a spiral electrode until the pattern becomes reassuring or until intervention for a nonreassuring pattern is indicated. Warning patterns include the following:

- Progressive increase/decrease or shift in baseline FHR
- Tachycardia of 160 bpm or more than 30 bpm from previous baseline
- Decreasing baseline variability without any identified cause (e.g., narcotics)

Nonreassuring Fetal Heart Rate Patterns and Interventions

Intervention for nonreassuring or worrisome FHR patterns (Figure 7-2) should be done using a step-by-step approach, and one should proceed to the next step only if the pattern is uncorrected.

Criteria for reassuring variable decelerations (Freeman, Garite, and Nageotte, 1991):

1. Last no more than 30 to 45 seconds
2. Have a rapid return to baseline (no evidence of a late component/slow return)
3. Baseline rate is not increasing
4. Variability is not decreasing

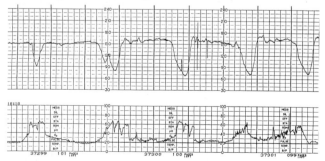

Figure 7-2
Suspicious FHR pattern of variable decelerations must be continually evaluated against criteria for a reassuring pattern.

Nonreassuring Fetal Heart Rate Patterns	Intervention
Severe variable deceleration: FHR below 70 bpm or 60 bpm below baseline, lasting longer than 60 seconds with any of the following: Rising baseline FHR Decreasing variability Slow return to baseline "Overshoot" without variability	With severe variable deceleration: Change maternal position Perform vaginal or speculum examination, or both Discontinue oxytocin if infusing (consider tocolysis) Administer oxygen at 8 to 10 L/min at 100% by snug face mask Amnioinfusion may be considered Termination of labor should be considered if pattern cannot be corrected enough to meet criteria of mild deceleration
Late decelerations of any magnitude, more serious if associated with decreasing variability or rising baseline	Intervene in step-by-step approach, proceeding to next step if pattern is uncorrected Place patient in lateral position Lower head of bed Increase rate of maintenance IV infusion

Purpose	Rationale
To relieve pressure on the umbilical cord	Improves umbilical and utero-placental blood flow
To rule out a prolapsed cord	Continue other interventions or set up for a cesarean delivery if cord is prolapsed
To reduce repetitive pressure on cord and decrease uterine hyperstimulation	Discontinue exogenous source of uterine stimulation
To promote maternal hyperoxia	Increases available oxygen to the fetus
To relieve pressure on the umbilical cord by adding fluid to "cushion" cord	Correct oligohydramnios
To decrease stress/hypoxia on fetus	Fetal position, stage of labor, dilatation, and effacement need to be considered in continuance of labor in the presence of a nonreassuring FHR pattern
To correct supine hypotension	Removes the weight of the fetus from the inferior vena cava, which then allows better blood return to the heart, increasing maternal cardiac output and subsequently blood pressure
To correct maternal hypotension	Diminishes pooling of blood in extremities and increases circulating volume
To correct maternal hypotension and reverse dehydration	Increases circulating blood volume

Nonreassuring Fetal Heart Rate Patterns	Intervention
	Discontinue oxytocin if infusing (consider tocolysis) (do this first if uterine hyperstimulation is present)
	Administer oxygen at 8 to 10 L/min at 100% by snug face mask
	Stimulate fetal scalp or give sound stimulation
Absence of variability	Correct identifiable cause
Prolonged deceleration	As above
Severe bradycardia	As above
Sinusoidal	As above

Purpose	Rationale
To reduce uterine activity	Decreases strength and frequency of uterine contractions, which can improve uteroplacental blood flow
To promote maternal hyperoxia	Increases fetal oxygenation
To identify FHR reactivity and produce acceleration; gives indication of fetal oxygenation and pH	Indicates fetal well-being; if the fetus is able to produce accelerations, it shows ability to compensate; pH is generally >7.2
To determine if result of narcotic administration, position, uterine hyperstimulation, rapid descent, cord prolapse, or abruption	To determine if cause is reversible or changeable; document event, notify appropriate OB team members and, if warranted, prepare for immediate delivery

Other Methods of Assessment/Intervention

The primary hypothesis for intrapartum surveillance is the timely identification of and intervention for the hypoxic or acidotic fetus to prevent intrauterine death and decrease long-term neurologic damage and sequela (Yoon et al, 1993). To date, an optimal method to identify hypoxia/acidosis has not been identified. Studies show that most accurate assessments of fetal well-being and degree of asphyxia are best determined when EFM is used in conjunction with other tools. Some tools of assessment are used during the intrapartum period and others after delivery. All help to reconstruct hypoxic episodes and to ascertain the degree of asphyxia of the neonate.

Fetal Heart Rate Response to Stimulation

Stimulation of the fetus to elicit an acceleration of FHR for at least 15 seconds has been reported as an alternative to scalp pH testing, a discussion of which is found in the next section. Several studies have correlated the fetal scalp pH with the FHR response to a stimulus and have attested to the efficacy of these mechanisms. Stimulation methods include the following:

1. *Scalp stimulation:* Digital pressure of the scalp for a 15-second period, followed by application of an atraumatic Allis clamp to the scalp for 15 seconds
2. *Sound stimulation:* Vibroacoustic stimulation by placing an artificial larynx on the maternal abdomen over the fetal head.

The rationale for use of these mechanisms is that if an acceleration of 15 bpm for 15 seconds occurs with the stimulation, one can assume that the fetal pH is normal. Studies have shown that no less than 50% of stimulated fetuses will have an FHR acceleration, and this is highly predictive of fetal well-being and a pH of no less than 7.25. Of the fetuses that do not accelerate, about one half are not acidotic; therefore absence of an acceleration to the stimulus is not totally predictive of an abnormal pH, fetal acidosis, or fetal distress.

Fetal Blood Sampling for Acid-Base Monitoring

Fetal blood sampling (Figure 7-3) was first described by Saling in 1962 as a means of identifying fetal hypoxemia and acidosis. When the fetus is faced with hypoxia, metabolism changes from aerobic to anaerobic. This results in the production of lactic acid and a subsequent drop in pH. Therefore a decrease in blood pH becomes a measure of the degree of hypoxia.

Thus fetal scalp sampling was developed as a means of identifying the degree of fetal hypoxia at the time of testing. Studies show that many variables can lead to false elevations or drops in results. This form of assessment is not usually a standard of practice in all institutions unless opportunities exist for development of technique and proper equipment for testing is readily available on site. Samples are usually collected aerobically and in small amounts. If the samples are difficult to obtain or the drops of blood are slow forming, the results may show falsely elevated pH values. Fetal scalp sampling is invasive, and initiation of sampling usually requires repeated sampling every 15 to 30 minutes to monitor pH values.

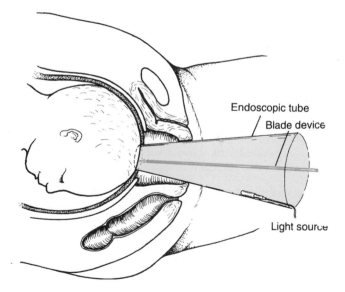

Endoscopic tube

Blade device

Light source

Figure 7-3
Schema of fetal blood sampling.

A small amount of fetal blood is obtained from the skin of the presenting part—usually the fetal scalp. To measure Po_2, Pco_2, and base deficit, a larger sample of fetal blood is required. Because these values do not provide enough additional information to warrant their measurement, and because blood gas values can vary so rapidly with transient circulatory changes, the use of fetal blood sampling during the intrapartum period is not routinely warranted. Measurements vary during different stages of labor. Various factors can influence pH during the intrapartum/predelivery period and make values disproportionate to the condition at birth. These factors are listed as follows:

1. Maternal acidosis or alkalosis
2. Laboratory errors in determination
3. Caput succedaneum ($\downarrow$ pH value)
4. Stage of labor
5. Time relationship of scalp sampling to uterine contractions
6. Influence of in utero treatment
7. Transience of the insult causing fetal acidosis (metabolic acidosis is less readily reversible than respiratory acidosis)
8. Contamination of sample with amniotic fluid ($\downarrow$ pH value) or room air ($\uparrow$ pH value)
9. Contamination with meconium

Interpretation of Values

The normal range of pH in an adult is 7.35 to 7.45. The average fetal range is 7.30 to 7.35, with values above 7.25 considered normal. A value between 7.20 and 7.25 is considered preacidotic, and the blood sample is usually repeated within 15 to 30 minutes to detect the possibility of a downward trend. A scalp blood pH of less than 7.15 is considered frank acidosis and indicates the need for some type of medical or surgical intervention.

Normal Fetal Scalp Values

pH	7.25-7.35
Po_2	18-22 mm Hg
Pco_2	40-50 mm Hg

Base deficit approximately 7 mEq/L

Anaerobic metabolism will occur in the fetus in the absence of oxygen, resulting in the production of lactic acid, which accumulates to lower the fetal pH and thus serves as an indirect measure of fetal oxygenation. When respiratory acidosis occurs in the fetus, as can occur with cord compression demonstrated by variable decelerations, the pH is low, the Pco_2 markedly elevated, and the base deficit usually unchanged. With metabolic acidosis caused by uteroplacental insufficiency and demonstrated by late decelerations, the pH is low, the Po_2 decreased, the Pco_2 mildly elevated, and the base deficit elevated (possibly exceeding 10 to 15 mEq/L).

Umbilical Cord Acid-Base Determination

A useful adjunct to the Apgar score in assessing the immediate condition of the newborn is to obtain a sample of cord blood. It may be helpful to rule out asphyxia in the presence of a low Apgar score. If metabolic acidosis is not present, then it is not likely that the low Apgar score is caused by intrapartum asphyxia.

The procedure consists of double clamping a 10 to 20 cm (approximately 4 to 8 inches) segment of the umbilical cord immediately after delivery of the infant. A specimen should be drawn with a 1-ml plastic syringe that has been flushed with heparin solution (1000 U/ml). Draw blood from the umbilical artery, or if that is not possible, from the umbilical vein. Separate syringes should be used if drawing blood from both the umbilical vein and umbilical artery. Normal values for cord blood are summarized as follows:

Normal Values for Umbilical Cord Blood

Cord blood	pH	Pco_2 mm Hg	Po_2 mm Hg	Bicarbonate mEq/L
Arterial	7.28	49.2	18.0	22.3
(range)	(7.15-7.43)	(31.1-74.3)	(3.8-33.8)	(13.3-27.5)
Venous	7.35	38.2	29.2	20.4
(range)	(7.24-7.49)	(23.2-49.2)	(15.4-48.2)	(15.9-24.7)

Continuous Monitoring of Fetal Oxygen Saturation by Pulse Oximetry

The use of pulse oximetry in labor and delivery is another method of assessment that is still undergoing study. Studies using the Nellcor fetal oxygen saturation monitor and fetal oxisensor (Nellcor Inc., Pleasanton, Calif.) have been done to determine the saturation readings of the fetus in comparison with the values of fetal blood sampling. In one study the oxisensor was positioned between the fetal cheek and uterine wall, which is less invasive and traumatic to the fetus. As a result of this study, it was concluded that fetal pulse oximetry corresponds satisfactorily with results from fetal blood analysis. In addition, the low degree of invasiveness and ability to provide continuous monitoring were considered to be the advantages of this method. The currently available sensor generates only a limited amount of signal time when used; however, when it is used in combination with electronic fetal heart rate monitoring, fetal pulse oximetry promises greatly improved detection of fetal hypoxia (Luttkus et al, 1995). Further studies and applications of this methodology are expected in the future.

Intervention for Fetal Distress
Amnioinfusion

Amnioinfusion is a procedure used to replace amniotic fluid with normal saline through the intrauterine pressure catheter. With the advent of amnioinfusion, fetal stress is decreased and the chances for a vaginal delivery are increased (Wallerstedt et al, 1994). Amnioinfusion is an effective technique used to reduce variable decelerations caused by cord compression and to reduce the incidence of meconium aspiration in the presence of thick meconium.

Patients with documented oligohydramnios (secondary to uteroplacental insufficiency, premature rupture of membranes, or postmaturity) are at risk for developing cord compression. Cord compression is evidenced by variable decelerations during labor. With oligohydramnios, when the uterus contracts the cord becomes more vulnerable to compression. Amnioinfusion replaces the "cushion" for the cord and relieves both the frequency and intensity of variable decelerations.

Another indication for amnioinfusion is the presence of moderate to thick ("pea soup") **meconium.** The presence or absence of meconium is now known to be a reliable indicator of the amount of fetal stress during labor (Berkus et al, 1994). It is estimated that 12% of all fetuses pass meconium before delivery. At approximately 36 weeks gestation, the fetus excretes motilin into the intestine, which facilitates peristalsis. Therefore the presence of meconium before 36 weeks gestation is unusual. In the presence of fetal hypoxia the anal sphincter relaxes and intestinal peristalsis increases, facilitating the passage of meconium in utero. Many fetuses who have meconium in their amniotic fluid at delivery do not show signs of hypoxia. However, the passage of meconium late in labor in association with fetal heart rate abnormalities has been shown to be a warning sign of possible fetal distress. The asphyxiated fetus gasps in utero and inhales meconium into the large airways. If meconium is not removed from these airways at birth (before the neonate's first breaths), the meconium is pulled into the distal airways and air is trapped in the alveoli, resulting in inadequate airway exchange (meconium aspiration syndrome).

Intrapartum patients with meconium present are considered to be high risk, and the FHR pattern needs to be continually assessed, with timely and appropriate interventions performed if nonreassuring patterns are identified. The purpose of amnioinfusion in the presence of moderate to thick meconium is to dilute and flush out the meconium. Studies show that when amnioinfusion has been used for the presence of meconium, Apgar scores are higher, the incidence of operative delivery is decreased, and less meconium is visualized below the vocal cords during intubation and suctioning (Wallerstedt et al, 1994).

To ensure that meconium is not aspirated by the neonate, special care should be taken during the delivery process. The nasopharynx and oropharynx should be suctioned immediately as the head is being delivered. The mother may need to be instructed to blow repetitively to refrain from pushing to allow for suctioning to occur before the neonate takes its first breath. Following delivery the neonate should be subject to endotracheal intubation and tracheal suctioning until the meconium is cleared. All of these procedures should be clearly described in the patient's record by the person performing them.

Saline has been found to be the replacement fluid most resembling amniotic fluid. However, more studies need to be done to address concerns about fetal electrolyte status in relation to amnioinfusion. One risk to this intervention is the potential for iatrogenic polyhydramnios. It is critical to accurately assess fluid output during amnioinfusion and to monitor for increases in uterine resting tone. Infusion pumps must be used to deliver the amnioinfusion solution. Documentation of total amount administered and any other complications that occur is imperative. Placental detachment may be the result of overdistention of the uterus secondary to iatrogenic polyhydramnios.

Theoretically, in the presence of abruptio placentae, the risk of fluid emboli is increased with the use of amnioinfusion. Umbilical cord prolapse with amnioinfusion is another possible concern if the presenting part is not engaged in the pelvic inlet. The temperature of the saline solution used for amnioinfusion is generally at room temperature for term infants or warmed to body temperature only by blood warmer if the fetus is preterm. Amnioinfusion solution should **never** be warmed in the microwave.

Indications

1. Laboring preterm patients with premature rupture of the membranes
2. Patients with otherwise uncorrectable variable decelerations during labor
3. Known cases of significant oligohydramnios at term when undergoing induction of labor
4. Presence of moderate to thick ("pea soup") meconium

Equipment and supplies

1. 1000 ml/normal saline solution (at room temperature)
2. Internal uterine catheter equipment, preferably with a double lumen or amnioport
3. Intravenous extension tubing with twin sites or arterial line (12 inches) and a four-way stopcock if needed
4. Volumetric infusion pump and tubing
5. Blood warmer or blood fluid warming set (optional)

NOTE: When the fetus is preterm and the procedure is being done prophylactically, a volumetric infusion pump and warming unit or normal saline warmed to body temperature (98.6° F) should be used.

Preprocedure

1. Place patient in left lateral position
2. Administer 100% oxygen by snug face mask 8 to 10 L/min if ordered by the physician
3. Continuously monitor the patient

Procedure

After the intrauterine catheter is inserted:
1. Connect the extension tubing, which has been prefilled with sterile distilled water (to prevent saline corrosion of the transducer),

between the three-way stopcock (connected to the pressure transducer) and the intrauterine catheter or follow the manufacturer's
instructions for an intrauterine catheter with a double lumen or
amnioport
2. Attach intravenous tubing to the bottle of room temperature normal saline
3. Attach the 18-gauge needle to the intravenous tubing connected
to the saline and insert the needle into the side port of the extension tubing just above the connection to the intrauterine catheter
or insert the IV tubing into the amnioport
4. Initiate the flow of normal saline solution and instill 15 to 20
ml/min until variable decelerations are resolved or start the infusion at 600 ml/hr (10 ml/min), then decrease to 150 to 20 ml/hr
as indicated by fetal response. This can be achieved when the
saline bottle is 3 to 4 feet above the level of the intrauterine
catheter tip and when the intravenous control device is wide
open, or this can be done by administering the solution through
a volumetric infusion pump
   a. When variable decelerations diminish or resolve, add an additional 250 ml of normal saline to promote a continuing variable deceleration-free FHR pattern
   b. If variable decelerations are not relieved after infusion of 800
to 1000 ml of normal saline solution, then procedure may be
discontinued and alternate interventions performed

Be aware that the recorded resting tone during amnioinfusion
will appear higher than normal, about 35 to 40 mm Hg, because of
resistance to outflow through the tiny holes in the tip of the catheter.
The true resting tone can be checked easily by shutting off the infusion.

Patient care

Care of the patient undergoing amnioinfusion includes the following:
1. Stop the infusion periodically, approximately every 30 minutes,
to note the baseline uterine pressure. Notify the physician if the
resting tone is greater than 25 mm Hg to evaluate continuation of
the procedure
2. Change the underpads frequently to ensure patient comfort. This
is necessary because of the increase in vaginal fluid leakage.

Tocolysis Therapy for Abnormal Fetal Heart Rate Patterns (Intrauterine Resuscitation)

Although tocolytic therapy is routinely used to prevent and manage preterm labor, it can be used as an adjunct to other interventions in the management of fetal distress. When the fetus is exhibiting signs of acute distress with concomitant increased uterine activity that is not responsive to position change and discontinuance of the oxytocin infusion, the administration of an intravenous injection of terbutaline of 0.125 to 0.250 mg can be administered while preparation for immediate delivery is in process. A cesarean delivery may be performed if the abnormal FHR pattern persists and the fetus cannot be safely delivered vaginally. Conversely, if the FHR pattern improves, then the patient may be allowed to continue labor. Terbutaline, which has a shorter time of onset, is preferred to magnesium sulfate, which has a longer time of onset of 10 to 15 minutes. If the patient delivers shortly after the administration of terbutaline, there is a risk of uterine atony and postpartum hemorrhage. Therefore appropriate preparations should be made if delivery appears imminent.

NOTE: A protocol for the management of preterm labor that describes the use of tocolytics for patients meeting the criteria for the diagnosis of preterm labor can be found in Appendix C.

Antepartum Monitoring

Evaluation of fetal well-being and maturity is essential in the management of high-risk pregnancy. Generally, routine fetal surveillance through antepartum monitoring and testing is not initiated until a practitioner intervenes in the event of a nonreassuring sign. Therefore the gestational age parameters to begin fetal surveillance vary from institution to institution and depend on the level of care given, that is whether the facility delivers primary or tertiary care and the availability for neonatal support in the nursery.

This chapter provides information on biophysical assessment (including ultrasound, the biophysical profile, and daily fetal movement count) and on biochemical assessment (including amniocentesis, percutaneous umbilical blood sampling, and chorionic villus sampling). The procedures for nonstress and contraction stress testing and an overview of other fetal assessment parameters are reviewed as well.

Ultrasound

Ultrasound diagnosis has many uses in obstetrics, the most common of which are diagnosis of early pregnancy; assessment of fetal gestational age ascertained by measurement of the fetal cranial biparietal diameter; measurement of amount of amniotic fluid; visualization of fetal heart and breathing movements; detection of neural tube defects, renal abnormalities, skeletal abnormalities, and cardiac anomalies; placental localization and determination of volumetric growth; identification of multiple gestation; detection of certain anomalies such as anencephaly and hydrocephaly; confirmation of fetal lie, position, and presenting part; and diagnosis of molar pregnancy, adnexal tumors such as corpus luteum cyst of pregnancy, ectopic pregnancy, and fetal death. Ultrasonic guidance for amniocentesis has become routine. This section presents a short background of ultrasound and its biophysical principles as well as examples of ultrasound uses.

Background

Experiments using high-frequency sound waves date back to the 1880s, but it was not until World War I that principles of ultrasound were applied to naval science. Most of us are familiar with the term *sonar* (sound navigation and ranging), which refers to the use of high-frequency sound or ultrasound from a ship on the water's surface to detect submerged submarines. The sonar operator of a surface ship would direct a beam of sound into the depths. Upon striking the submerged submarine an echo would return to the sonar source. Based on the time it took for the echo to return after the original sound left the instrument, the operator could calculate the distance and location of that submarine.

Another use of ultrasound that developed during the wartime years was in the detection of flaws in metals used for industrial purposes.

The use of ultrasound in medicine was first reported in the late 1940s in the detection of cranial abnormalities, intracranial tumors, and gallstones. Ultrasound diagnosis is commonly used now to detect tumors, to locate anatomical structures, and to assess cardiac function by means of a process known as echocardiography.

Dr. Ian Donald of Glasgow, Scotland, pioneered the use of diagnostic ultrasound in obstetrics and gynecology and first reported the detection of gynecologic neoplasms in 1958. Since then, Dr. Donald and several other investigators have reported its use in obstetrics, and ultrasound examination is now commonplace in antenatal diagnosis of the fetal condition.

Biophysical Principles

Ultrasound is the use of those sound waves beyond the range of human hearing. Sound is measured in Hertz, which denotes cycles per second. The audible range of hearing is from 20 to 20,000 Hz (Hertz). Ultrasound used for obstetric diagnosis is generally 2.25 M Hz (2.25 mega Hertz), although the range for diagnostic ultrasound is from 1 M Hz to 15 M Hz. The following list contrasts sound frequency with various descriptive uses.

Audible range
20 Hz
60 Hz Boom of a bass drum

84	Hz Bass voice
256	Hz Middle C on piano
1,125	Hz Soprano voice
20,000	Hz

Inaudible

| 50,000 | Hz Ultrasonic cleaners |

Diagnostic ultrasound

1,000,000	Hz
2,250,000	Hz Obstetric diagnosis
15,000,000	Hz

Ultrasound used in diagnostic work is generated by a transducer, a device that converts energy from one form to another. The ultrasound is produced by the ringing of a crystal wafer of a material having piezoelectric properties. The word *piezoelectric* is derived from the German language and literally translates as "pressure electric." Crystalline quartz, lithium sulfate, lead zirconate, and barium titanate have piezoelectric properties—the ability to convert mechanical pressure into electrical energy and vice versa. The crystal is struck electrically to produce a mechanical pulse of 2.25 M Hz. When ultrasound produced by the crystal transverses an object at a 90° angle, or is perpendicular to it, the echoes returning to the crystal probe are recorded as dots of light on a cathode ray oscilloscope screen. The intensity and brightness of the dots correspond to the density and acoustic impedance or resistance met by the searching beam of sound at the various tissue interfaces. By moving the transducer in a specific scanning motion, the dots from each tissue interface coalesce to trace the anatomical outline of that region. The display is then photographed for a permanent record (Figure 8-1).

Visualization of the fetus by ultrasonography can be achieved through a hand-held device placed on the patient's abdomen as well as through a transvaginal approach most commonly done early in gestation.

Examples of Ultrasonography

Usually an abdominal and pelvic examination can determine fetal lie. In an obese patient or one who is difficult to examine it is sometimes impossible to determine whether the fetus is in a breech or vertex presentation or a transverse lie. Ultrasound examination can readily determine fetal presentation (Figures 8-2, 8-3, 8-4, and 8-5).

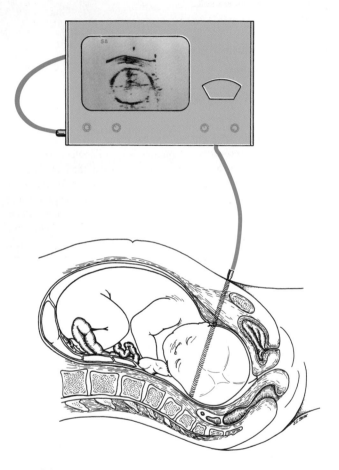

Figure 8-1
The fetal head is displayed on the screen when the ultrasound transducer is perpendicular to fetal BPD. The biparietal diameter (BPD) is determined by measuring distance between proximal and distal skull echoes.

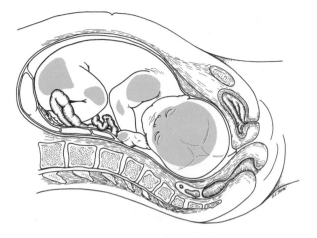

Figure 8-2
Schema of longitudinal section illustrates fetal head, body, and extremity in sonogram.

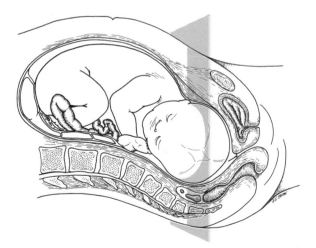

Figure 8-3
Schema of transverse section illustrates fetal head in sonogram.

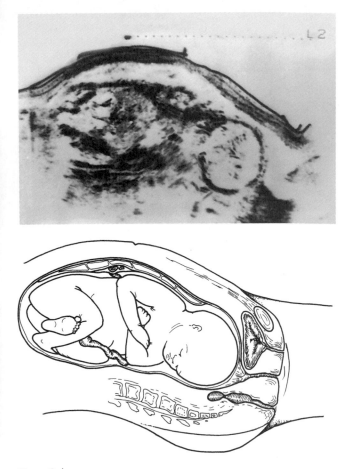

Figure 8-4
Sonogram contrasted with schema of cephalic presentation in longitudinal section.

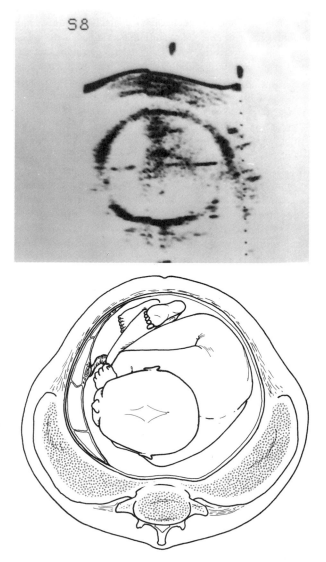

Figure 8-5
Sonogram contrasted with schema of cephalic presentation in transverse section.

Safety

Diagnostic ultrasound is apparently harmless. No detrimental effects have been observed to date on the fetus or mother either histologically, functionally, or embryologically in experimental work. Diagnostic ultrasound's greatest value to obstetrics lies in the fact that it allows the possibility of repeated examinations during pregnancy and the acquisition of valuable information without jeopardizing the fetus or the mother. This contrasts with ionizing radiation, which cannot be used repeatedly because of the past occurrence of malignant disease in children who had been irradiated in utero.

An ordinary x-ray film is a shadow picture in which the body area is placed between the x-ray tube and the photographic plate or screen. All areas and all thicknesses are irradiated simultaneously. This contrasts with ultrasound, in which the sound waves and the receiving point are on the same side of the body. Only a pencil-like volume of the body is insonated at any one time.

The widespread acceptance of ultrasound diagnosis in obstetrics is based on the absence of detrimental effects to the fetus and mother, the safety or repeated examinations, and the convenience of its being done on an outpatient basis.

Indications

The use of ultrasound in obstetrics is indicated for the following:
1. Diagnosis of early pregnancy
2. Appraisal of fetal growth through serial determinations of the biparietal diameter
3. Localization of the placenta
4. Identification of multiple gestation
5. Diagnosis of molar pregnancy
6. Placental volumetric growth
7. Detection of certain fetal abnormalities such as anecephaly (Figure 8-6) and hydrocephaly
8. Detection of hydramnios and oligohydramnios
9. Diagnosis of fetal death (Figure 8-7)
10. Confirmation of fetal lie, position, and presenting part
11. Identification of compound presentation
12. Guidance for amniocentesis
13. Fetal breathing movements
14. Fetal movement
15. Fetal tone
16. Amniotic fluid index

Ultrasound can also be used to detect fetal cardiac anomalies through echocardiography.

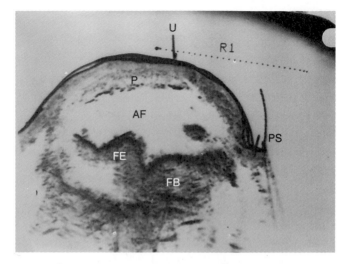

Figure 8-6
Anencephaly. Longitudinal section 1 cm to right of midline
(R1). Fetal body *(FB)* and fetal extremity *(FE)* can be seen.
Note absence of fetal head and concurrent hydramnios with
large area filled with amniotic fluid *(AF)*.

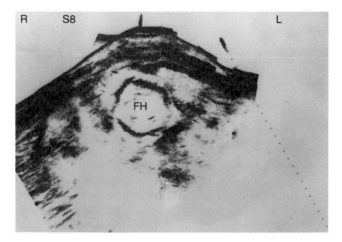

Figure 8-7
Fetal death. Transverse section 8 cm above pubic symphysis
(S8). Outline of fetal head is irregular due to overlapping of
cranial bones.

Biophysical Profile

Description

The biophysical profile is a noninvasive, dynamic assessment of the fetus and fetal environment. The assessment is performed using real-time ultrasound and the electronic fetal heart rate monitor. Parameters measured in this evaluation include:

1. Fetal breathing movements (FBM)
2. Fetal movement (FM)
3. Fetal tone (FT)*
4. Amniotic fluid index (AFI)*
5. Nonstress test (NST)*

Clinical Significance

Fetal heart rate reactivity, fetal movements, fetal breathing movements, and fetal tone are acute biophysical markers and are believed to be initiated and regulated by complex, integrated mechanisms of the fetal CNS. Normal biophysical activity is indirect evidence that the portion of the CNS that controls that specific activity is intact. However, the absence of biophysical activities is difficult to interpret since it may reflect pathologic depression or normal fetal periodicity.

The measurement of the amniotic fluid index (AFI) is a marker of chronic fetal condition.

Investigators have shown an inverse relationship between NST and AFI findings. The lower the AFI, the greater the incidence of nonreactive tests, decelerations, and perinatal morbidity and mortality.

Therefore since the development of the four-quadrant AFI measurement, this technique and the NST have been used together with increasing frequency to identify the fetus at risk for complications related to decreased amniotic fluid.

*Most indicative of fetal well-being

Interpretation

Biophysical profile scoring

Biophysical Variable	Normal (Score = 2)	Abnormal (Score = 0)
Fetal breathing movements (FBM)	At least one episode of FBM of at least 30 sec duration in 30-min observation	Absent FBM or no episode of ≥30 sec in 30 min
Gross body movements (FM)	At least three discrete body/limb movements in 30 min (episodes of active continuous movement considered as a single movement)	Two or fewer episodes of body/limb movements in 30 min
Fetal tone (FT)	At least one episode of active extension with return to flexion of fetal limb(s) or trunk; opening and closing of hand considered normal tone	Either slow extension with return to partial flexion or movement of limb in full extension or absence of fetal movement
Amniotic fluid index (AFI) (varies by gestational age)	Sum total of measurements in cm from each quadrant is 5.1 to 24 cm (low normal is 5.1 to 9.9 cm)	Sum total of measurements in cm from each quadrant is ≤5 cm or >24 cm
Nonstress test (NST)	Reactive—two or more episodes of FHR acceleration ≥15 bpm ≥15 sec	Nonreactive

The Biophysical Profile should be recorded on the patient's progress sheet. An example of a biophysical profile scoring format follows.

Parameter	Score
Fetal Breathing Movements (FBM)	
Fetal Movement (FM)	
Fetal Tone (FT)	
Amniotic Fluid Index (AFI)	
Nonstress Test (NST)	
	TOTAL: _____

Management

Score	Action
8-10	Equivalent to reactive NST; indicates fetus at minimal risk for fetal death or damage within 1 week
4-6	If pulmonary maturity is favorable, deliver; if not, repeat test in 24 hours; if score persists, deliver if maturity is certain; otherwise, treat with corticosteroids to promote pulmonary maturity and deliver in 48 hours. Incidence of perinatal complications is higher.
0-2	Evaluate for delivery; has been associated with a perinatal mortality rate of 60% or greater (Gegor and Paine, 1992)

Amniotic Fluid Index Measurement

Procedure	Rationale
Assist patient into the low semi-Fowler's position	To avoid hypotension
	To have enough exposure of the abdomen for placement of ultrasound transducer on the appropriate area of the abdomen
Divide the uterus into four equal quadrants. At term, using the umbilicus, draw an imaginary line across the vertical axis and using the linea negra, draw an imaginary longitudinal line up and down the abdomen	To divide abdomen into four equal quadrants

Procedure	Rationale
Holding the ultrasound transducer in the longitudinal plane and perpendicular to the floor, view each quadrant separately. Using calipers, measure the deepest pocket of fluid in each quadrant. Exclude umbilical cord and fetal parts from measurements	By appropriate placement of the transducer, measuring fluid from an adjacent quadrant is avoided. In addition, keeping the transducer perpendicular avoids an oblique measurement of the pockets, which would result in a falsely increased apparent size of the pocket (Figure 8-8).
Add all values obtained	To determine the amniotic fluid index

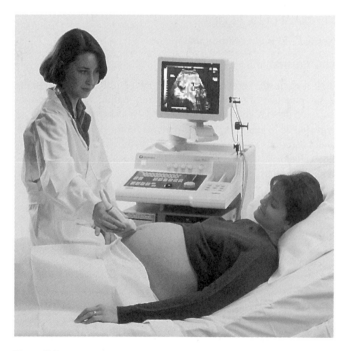

Figure 8-8
Nurse performing Amniotic Fluid Index (AFI) measurement with the Aloka 650CL ultrasound.
(Courtesy Corometrics Medical Systems, Inc., Wallingford, Conn.)

AFI Values

>24 cm	Increased
10-24 cm	Normal
5.1-9.9 cm	Low Normal
≤5 cm	Decreased

Interpretation
Increased AFI(>24 cm)

Increased AFI is an indication for antepartum testing, including serial AFI measurements at least weekly. A complete ultrasound examination should be conducted to evaluate for associated fetal and placental anomalies as well as for workup of polyhydramnios, including infection, diabetes, and isoimmunization.

Normal AFI (10-24 cm)

Normal AFI is a reassuring finding during fetal testing.

Low normal AFI (5.1-9.9 cm)

Low normal AFI should be evaluated taking into consideration the gestational age of the fetus. Since amniotic fluid volume peaks at 34 to 35 weeks gestation, an AFI of less than 10 cm should be reevaluated by additional measurements for the presence of associated conditions such as intrauterine growth retardation. A borderline value of 5.1 cm to 7 cm should be reevaluated every 3 to 4 days if all other findings remain normal.

Decreased AFI (≤5 cm)

Decreased AFI values of 5 cm or less in a patient at term or postterm indicate the need to deliver the fetus. When no amniotic fluid is found, a complete ultrasound examination should be conducted to rule out fetal anomalies. Rupture of the membranes may be a cause for decreased or absent amniotic fluid.

Fetal Movement

Various investigators have reported a marked decrease in fetal movement before an episode of fetal distress or fetal death. It is interesting to note that now there is scientific evidence for a concept believed, practiced, and relied on by generations midwives and mothers.

Generally, the number of fetal movements decreases from early to late pregnancy in normal gestation. In pregnancies complicated by uteroplacental insufficiency, there is a marked decrease in daily fetal movement count (DFMC), and a precipitous fall occurs in the period immediately preceding fetal death. The advantages of fetal movement counting are that it is inexpensive, continuously available away from the clinical area, and relatively simple for the patient to do, although accuracy and reliability are variable.

Parameters for normal daily fetal movement counts or "kick counts" vary slightly in practice from 3 to 10 movements in 1 hour to 3 in 30 minutes. Procedure varies with time of day, reference to mealtime (just after eating), maternal position (lateral), and with hydration (water or juice). The patient is instructed to "be quiet with herself," be relaxed but awake, have an empty bladder, place her hands on her abdomen, and focus on the baby's movements. When the patient is instructed to do kick counts, it is often helpful to use palpation and verify with the patient what sensations can be interpreted as fetal movements. Patients should continue to be aware of fetal movements and report the hourly observations if she perceives decreased fetal movement. It is important to note that fetal movement can occur without maternal recognition (based on studies that show maternal perception is only 40% of actual fetal movement at term [Stanco, 1993]). An NST is often performed if only one or two movements are felt within a 1-hour period. Amniotic fluid indexing may also be done. If the NST is reactive, further testing may not be done unless there are some other risk factors of if the patient again perceives a decrease in fetal movement. A nonreactive NST would be followed as soon as possible by a biophysical profile (BPP) or contraction stress test (CST).

Kick Count Methodology
Patient instructions

Six Steps: How to Use Your Counting Log

1. Count movements anytime between 7:00 PM and 11:00 PM.
2. After you eat, lie down on your left or right side.
3. Mark down the **date** and **start time** on your log.
4. Place your hands over your abdomen and pay close attention to your baby's movements.
5. Every time your baby moves **or** kicks mark one of the boxes.
6. When the baby has moved **or** kicked 10 times write down the **stop time** on your log.

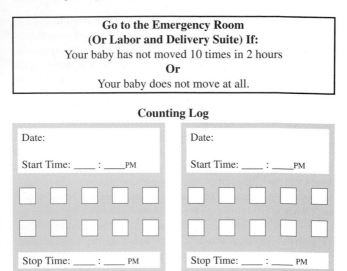

**Go to the Emergency Room
(Or Labor and Delivery Suite) If:**
Your baby has not moved 10 times in 2 hours
Or
Your baby does not move at all.

Counting Log

Date:	Date:
Start Time: ____ : ____PM	Start Time: ____ : ____PM
☐ ☐ ☐ ☐ ☐	☐ ☐ ☐ ☐ ☐
☐ ☐ ☐ ☐ ☐	☐ ☐ ☐ ☐ ☐
Stop Time: ____ : ____ PM	Stop Time: ____ : ____ PM

Day 1   Day 2

Developed by the Women's Hospital Antepartum Testing Unit LAC-USC Medical Center, Los Angeles, Calif. Courtesy of Yolanda Rabello, RNC, CCRN.

Fetoscopy

Fetoscopy is the direct visualization of the fetus with an endoscope inserted into the amniotic cavity through the maternal abdomen. The procedure is done to directly view portions of the fetal anatomy in patients whose fetuses are at risk for specifically suspected abnormalities and for Ellis-van Creveld syndrome, an autosomal recessive trait in which affected infants have short limbs, cardiac abnormalities, and always exhibit polydactyly. This technique has also been used for directing skin biopsies and less frequently to obtain fetal blood in the diagnosis of fetal hemoglobinopathies. Fetoscopy may be used as an adjunct to laser ablation of connecting vessels in twin–twin transfusion syndrome. Real-time ultrasound is used during the procedure to guide the fetoscope to an appropriate area for viewing or blood sampling.

Fetoscopy is generally performed at 18 weeks of gestation. Complications of this procedure are spontaneous abortion, preterm delivery, leakage of amniotic fluid, amnionitis, and intrauterine fetal death.

An analgesic may be given to the patient to limit fetal movement during the procedure. Postprocedure care includes monitoring of vital signs, administration of anti-Rh globulin as indicated, and teaching patients to report any pain, bleeding, amniotic fluid loss, or fever.

Amnioscopy

Amnioscopy is the direct visualization of amniotic fluid through the fetal membranes with a cone-shaped hollow tube when the cervix is sufficiently dilated. It is done to identify meconium staining of the amniotic fluid, which results from an episode of fetal hypoxia causing relaxation of the anal sphincter and an increase in fetal peristalsis.

Amnioscopy is of value in postdate pregnancies when the possibility of postmature syndrome exists.

The amnioscope is also used to visualize the presenting part after rupture of membranes to obtain a fetal blood sample for blood gas analysis. The procedure is performed with the patient in lithotomy position and takes approximately 10 minutes. The patient should be instructed that dilation of the cervix from the endoscope may cause some discomfort and menstrual-type cramping may continue for some time after the procedure is completed.

Amniography

Amniography is the injection of radiopaque agents into the amniotic sac to identify hydramnios, oligohydramnios, placenta previa, the soft tissue silhouette of the fetus, and—after a few hours of swallowing—the fetal gastrointestinal tract. Meconium staining of the amniotic fluid may follow this procedure, especially if the fetus is approaching term. However, this is not specifically indicative of fetal distress. Because ultrasonography provides most of the information that amniography does without the use of ionizing radiation or injection into the amniotic sac, amniography is rarely done.

Magnetic Resonance Imaging

Magnetic resonance imaging (MRI) is a noninvasive tool that provides excellent visualization of soft tissue. This technique can be used to evaluate fetal structures, placenta position and density, amniotic fluid quantity, maternal structures and soft tissue, and meta-

bolic or functional malformations. The time required for the procedure is rather lengthy, from 20 to 60 minutes, during which time the
patient must be very still. Although the information gleaned from
this procedure is very specific, broad usage is limited because of the
time involved, fetal movement, and other acceptable alternatives to
obtain similar information.

Computed Tomography

Computed tomography (CT scan) pelvimetry is used occasionally to
assess the anatomic pelvis in anticipation of a vaginal breech delivery.

Radiography

Radiologic assessment for fetal size, maturity, and placental localization is seldom done since the advent of ultrasound diagnosis. In
recent years there has been growing concern over the use of ionizing radiation because of potential carcinogenic, teratogenic, and mu-
tagenic effects. The scope of these risks has yet to be clearly identified.

A simple roentgenogram of the abdomen and pelvis after 16
weeks gestation will most often identify fetal skeletal parts. During
the second half of pregnancy the number of fetuses can be seen in a
multiple gestation. Anencephaly and hydrocephaly can be identified during the third trimester. There is some correlation between
fetal age and the time of appearance of lower limb ossification centers, but this varies with fetal sex and weight.

Radiography is essentially only done in nonobstetrical applications such as for an IVP (intravenous pyelogram) or trauma because ultrasound can provide the necessary information regarding
the fetus.

Amniocentesis

Amniocentesis, the removal of fluid from the amniotic cavity by
needle puncture (Figure 8-9), was described in the early 1950s by
Bevis (1952), who noted the varying degrees of bile pigments in
amniotic fluid discovered while assessing Rh-isoimmunized pregnancies. Since then, the use of amniocentesis has become a standard tool in the assessment of fetal well-being and maturity and in
the diagnosis of genetic defects.

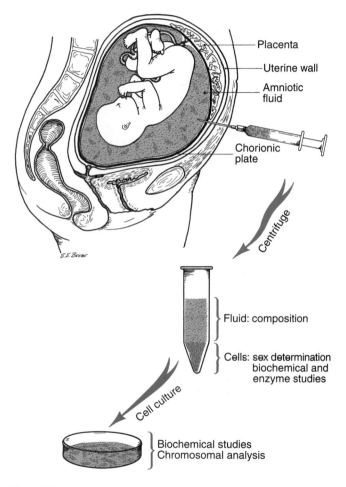

Placenta
Uterine wall
Amniotic fluid
Chorionic plate
Centrifuge

Fluid: composition
Cells: sex determination biochemical and enzyme studies

Cell culture

Biochemical studies
Chromosomal analysis

Figure 8-9
Amniocentesis. Amniotic fluid is aspirated with a sterile syringe. Sample is centrifuged to separate cells and fluid. A variety of tests can be done.

An amniocentesis is the penetration of the amniotic cavity through the abdominal and uterine wall for the purpose of withdrawing fluid for examination. The procedure is performed by insertion of a 20 to 22 gauge spiral-type needle transabdominally to aspirate 5 to 20 ml of amniotic fluid.

When genetic problems are suspected, amniocentesis is performed before 16 weeks gestation. This permits time for karyotyping and biochemical studies to be completed before the time limit for having an elective abortion. If the parents are not amenable to elective abortion for an abnormal fetus, the amniocentesis may not be warranted.

Amniocentesis later in pregnancy is most often performed to assess fetal well-being and maturity. In cases of isoimmunization the procedure may be performed repeatedly to monitor the fetal condition. In high-risk pregnancies, such as those with maternal diabetes, amniocentesis may be performed to assess fetal lung maturity, indicating the most opportune time for delivery.

There are minimal risks to amniocentesis. Several researchers have reported that less than 0.5% of all amniocentesis procedures result in spontaneous abortion. Other risks include trauma to the fetus or to the placenta, bleeding, infection, premature labor, and Rh sensitization from fetal bleeding into the maternal circulation. Overall, however, the risk of amniocentesis to the mother or the fetus is generally accepted to be in the range of 0.5%. This is markedly reduced partially because of the use of ultrasonographic guidance during the procedure.

Before amniocentesis for any reason the physician informs the patient of specific risk factors. This verbal interaction is documented by a consent form. Although the wording varies from institution to institution, the forms are consistent in basic content. They include the following key points:

1. The risk factor to mother and fetus is approximately 0.5%
2. The culture of fetal cells may not be successful
3. Repeated amniocentesis may be required
4. Chromosome analysis, biochemical analysis, or both may not be successful
5. Normal chromosome results, normal biochemical results, or both do not eliminate the possibility that the child may have birth defects or mental retardation because of other disorders

Patient Care

The nurse has a key role in supporting the patient through the procedure of amniocentesis since patients approach it with a variety of feelings and questions. Initially the patient may wonder whether she should expose herself and her fetus to the risk of amniocentesis. She may use the results to decide if she will terminate an abnormal pregnancy. She may question the ramifications of continuing a pregnancy with an abnormal fetus, projecting her thoughts past delivery into the "quality of life" issue. The nurse can act as a support figure by being knowledgeable about the procedure, by answering questions factually, and by reinforcing explanations given by the physician.

During amniocentesis the nurse should stand by the side or at the head of the patient. The patient must remain quiet during the procedure and must be instructed not to touch the abdomen or drapes. Placing the patient's hands under her head serves as a reminder. Since most women are quite anxious when they see the length of the needle, they should be visually distracted or requested to close their eyes before needle entry. Patients who do not watch needle insertion usually report feeling only a sense of pressure on the abdomen.

Body proximity, eye contact, and touch by the nurse offer a sense of security and support. A damp washcloth on a perspiring forehead may be soothing. A nervous hand held by the nurse may be comforting. Anxious words and impromptu comments should be accepted by the nurse with a supportive attitude.

When the amniocentesis is completed, the patient should be observed for any untoward symptoms. If the patient feels faint, she should be assisted in turning to her left side. This will counteract any *supine hypotension* (caused by uterine pressure on the vena cava) by increasing venous return, blood pressure, and cardiac output. The patient's vital signs should be monitored postprocedure. The uterine fundus should be palpated at the same time to note fetal or uterine activity.

When the patient has fully recovered, she should be instructed to report any of the following to the physician: vaginal drainage, fetal hyperactivity or unusual quietness, uterine contractions, signs of infection such as fever or chills, abdominal pain, and vaginal bleeding.

Amniotic Fluid Analysis

Amniotic fluid derives mostly from fetal urine and secretions and contains fetal cells. The sample is centrifuged to separate the cells from the fluid.

Color

A bloody tap may result in cell growth failure and changes the level of other amniotic fluid constituents in the direction of predicting a less mature fetus.

A greenish tinged or a thick, dark-green sample indicates the presence of meconium. Aside from indicating a patent fetal anus, the presence of meconium is generally accepted to be associated with some degree of fetal hypoxia. However, the exact cause for the presence of meconium is not known, and it is often observed in the absence of hypoxia. The presence of meconium interferes with the reliability of other tests such as the L/S ratio and the bilirubin ΔOD.

Lecithin/sphingomyelin (L/S) ratio

Pulmonary surfactant primarily contains phospholipids. Surfactant acts as a surface detergent at the air-liquid interface of the alveoli, preventing their collapse at the end of an expiration. Without surfactant a neonate develops respiratory distress syndrome (RDS), a condition associated with immaturity in which the alveoli of the lung literally collapse with each expiration.

The L/S ratio assesses two phospholipids—lecithin and sphingomyelin—that comprise the largest part of the surfactant complex. Normally during gestation the sphingomyelin concentrations are greater than those of lecithin until about 26 weeks gestation. From 26 to 34 weeks gestation the concentration of lecithin to sphingomyelin is fairly equal, and therefore the L/S ratio is approximately 1:1. From 34 to 36 weeks gestation there is a sudden increase in lecithin and the ratio rapidly rises. It is generally accepted that a ratio of 2.0 or greater indicates pulmonary maturity and that respiratory distress syndrome (RDS) will rarely occur in the neonate. In a macrosomic fetus, as occurs in a diabetic gestation, the association between the L/S ratio and RDS is adversely affected. (See following discussion of Lung Profile.) The following interpretation is generally accepted:

L/S Ratio	Fetal Lung	Risk for RDS
>2.0	Mature	Minimal
1.50-2.0	Transitional zone	Moderate
<1.50	Immature	High

Some stressful conditions during pregnancy have been known to accelerate fetal lung maturity. They include preeclampsia, prolonged ruptured membranes, narcotic addiction, and intrauterine growth retardation. This acceleration may be a reflex fetal response to a hostile intrauterine environment. In contrast, conditions in which fetal lung maturity tends to be delayed include diabetes mellitus and fetal hemolytic disease.

Acceleration of fetal lung maturity has been achieved when the glucocorticoid betamethasone was injected into patients in whom premature delivery was anticipated. The fetal lung matured as reflected by a rise in the L/S ratio within 48 hours after initiating therapy.

The technique used to measure the L/S ratio by thin layer chromotography was developed by Gluck and associates (Gluck, 1971). To reduce laboratory time in performing the L/S ratio, the foam stability or "shake test" was introduced by Clements (1972) and coworkers. The "shake test" is based on the ability of surfactant to generate a stable foam when ethanol is added to the amniotic fluid specimen. Ethanol, isotonic saline, and amniotic fluid in measured amounts and varying dilutions are shaken together for 15 seconds. A ring of bubbles at the air-liquid interface at the proper dilution after 15 minutes indicates probable fetal lung maturity (Figure 8-10).

Measurement of the L/S ratio may be omitted when the "shake test" is positive because false-positive tests are rare. False-negative tests, however, are common and require awaiting the L/S ratio.

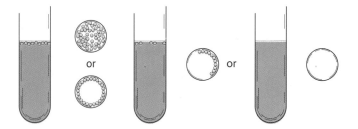

Positive foam test   Negative foam test

Figure 8-10
Clement's foam test (the shake test). For test to be positive, bubbles must be seen around entire circumference of tube.

Table 8-1   Various biochemical monitoring techniques*

Test	Results	Significance of Findings
Maternal blood		
Triple Marker Screening[†]		
Serum alphafetoprotein (AFP)	Low level	Possible Down Syndrome
β-hCG	High level	
Unconjugated estriol (E₃)	Low level	
Human placental lactogen	High levels	Large diabetic fetus; multiple gestation
	Low levels	Threatened abortion; IUGR; postmaturity
Alphafetoprotein	>40 ng/ml	Fetal neural tube defect
Coombs' test	Titer of 1:8 and rising	Significant isoimmunization
Amniocentesis		
Color	Meconium	Possible hypoxia
Lung Profile		Fetal lung maturity
L/S ratio	≥2.0	
PL	>50%	
PI	15-20%	
PG	2-10%	

Amniostat	PG ≥2 µg/ml	Fetal lung maturity
Disaturated phosphatidylcholine (DSPC)	≥500 µg/dL	
Shake test	Complete ring of bubbles after shaking at 1:2 dilution	
Foam stability index	≥47	
Creatinine	>2.0 mg/dl	Gestational age >36 weeks
Bilirubin (ΔOD 450)	<0.015	Gestational age >36 weeks; normal pregnancy
	High levels	Fetal hemolytic disease in isoimmunized pregnancies
Lipid cells	>10%	Gestational age >35 weeks
Alphafetoprotein	High levels after 15 weeks gestation	Open neural tube defect
Osmolality	Decline after 20 weeks gestation	Advancing nonspecific gestational age
Genetic disorders	Dependent on cultured cells for karyotype and enzymatic activity	
Sex-linked		
Chromosomal		
Metabolic		

*In an effort to summarize these studies in tabular form, generalizations have been made.
†From Benn, 1995 and Mooney, 1994.

Lung profile

The association between the L/S ratio and the incidence of respiratory distress syndrome does not always hold true in the diabetic gestation. RDS has been reported in neonates who had mature L/S ratios. The Lung Profile overcomes the problem of assessing lung maturity in the fetus of the diabetic and adds a parameter of security when interruption of pregnancy is contemplated.

The Lung Profile measures the interrelationships among the surfactant phospholipids: the lecithin/sphingomyelin (L/S) ratio, disaturated (acetone precipitated) lecithin (PL), phosphatidyl inositol (PI), and phosphatidyl glycerol (PG). Functional maturity of the lung occurs with the combination of these phospholipids. Phosphatidyl glycerol acts as a lung stabilizer, and when it is present in diabetic gestations with a mature L/S ratio, one can be confident that RDS will not occur.

Amniostat-FLM is an immunologic test with agglutination in the presence of phosphatidyl glycerol.

Amniotic fluid creatinine

There is a progressive rise in amniotic fluid creatinine values during the latter half of pregnancy, with a rapid rise near term. This is most likely due to an increased excretion of creatinine by the maturing fetal kidneys. A level of 2.0 mg/100 ml of amniotic fluid most often indicates fetal maturity and 36 or more weeks gestation. There are two cautions in the interpretation of this test: (1) the fetal lungs may be mature even when the creatinine is less than 2.0 mg/100 ml and (2) amniotic fluid creatinine may reflect an increased maternal plasma creatinine although the fetus is not mature. Therefore, it is unreliable to use amniotic fluid creatinine as the only component to assess fetal maturity.

Amniotic fluid bilirubin

During the second half of pregnancy the concentration of amniotic fluid bilirubin decreases until it virtually disappears during the last month of gestation. This measurement can be used to complement other laboratory values in assessing gestational age. However, it is not sensitive enough to be used alone for that purpose and has generally been replaced by the L/S ratio.

Amniotic fluid bilirubin is usually analyzed with a spectrophotometer measuring the optical density (OD) of the specimen against the characteristic absorption peak at 450 nm.* The value is usually expressed as ΔOD 450. It is important that the specimen of amniotic fluid not be exposed to light at any time for more than a few seconds, as this can invalidate the test. Amber glass specimen containers can be used, or clear test tubes can be covered with occlusive tape to protect the specimen from light.

In Rh-negative-sensitized pregnancies, as identified by maternal antibody titer (indirect Coombs' test), amniocentesis for bilirubin is one method of evaluating the severity of fetal hemolytic disease (Figure 8-11).

Percutaneous Umbilical Blood Sampling

Percutaneous umbilical blood sampling is achieved through the transabdominal insertion of a needle into a fetal umbilical vessel under ultrasound guidance. The ideal insertion point is near the placental insertion. Between 1 and 4 ml of blood are removed during the procedure and tested by the Kleihauer-Betke procedure to ensure that the specimen is fetal blood. The blood sample is used for determining karyotyping, direct Coombs', CBC, fetal blood type, blood gases, acid-base status for IUGR fetuses, detection of infection, and assessment and treatment of isoimmunization.

Complications are unusual and are due to blood leakage from the puncture site, fetal bradycardia, and chorioamnionitis (Bald et al, 1991) (Figure 8-12).

Chorionic Villus Sampling

Chorionic villus sampling (CVS) is the transcervical or transabdominal insertion of a needle into the fetal portion of the placenta to remove a small tissue specimen. The procedure is done between 10 and 12 weeks of gestation. The procedure is performed under real-time ultrasound visualization. The aspiration cannula and obturator traverse the cervical canal, and caution is exercised to avoid rupturing the amniotic sac. A transabdominal approach is an alternative to the transcervical technique. This procedure can be performed early in the first trimester to identify fetuses with genetic defects.

---

*In the Systeme International d'Unites (SI) nanometer (nm) replaces millimicron (mμ) as the designation for 10^{-9} meters.

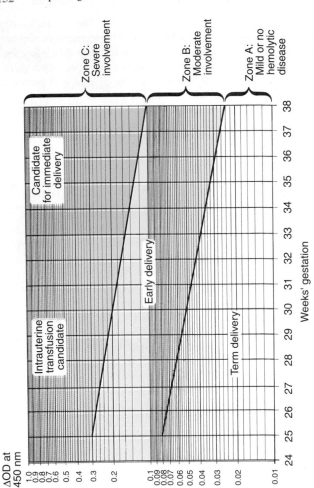

Figure 8-11
Prediction of severity of fetal hemolytic disease from amniotic fluid with management guidelines.

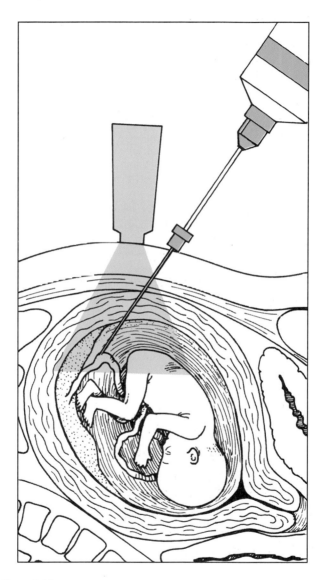

Figure 8-12

Technique for percutaneous umbilical blood sampling guided by ultrasound.

(From Bobak IM et al: *Maternity and gynecologic care: the nurse and the family,* ed 5, St. Louis, 1993, Mosby.)

Complications are rare after the procedure and include vaginal spotting or bleeding, spontaneous abortion, rupture of membranes, and chorioamnionitis. Rh immune globulin should be given to Rh negative women because of the possibility of fetomaternal hemorrhage, which could result in isoimmunization (Figure 8-13).

Nonstress and Stress Testing

The contraction stress test (CST), the nonstress test (NST), and fetal movement counts have been widely employed for the determination of fetal well-being.

Some indications for both the NST and the CST follow:
1. Suspected postmaturity (postdates ≥42 weeks)
2. Maternal diabetes mellitus
3. Chronic hypertension
4. Hypertensive disorders in pregnancy
5. Suspected and documented intrauterine growth retardation
6. Sickle cell disease
7. Maternal cyanotic heart disease
8. History of previous stillbirth
9. Blood group sensitization (isoimmunization)
10. Meconium-stained amniotic fluid (at amniocentesis)
11. Hyperthyroidism

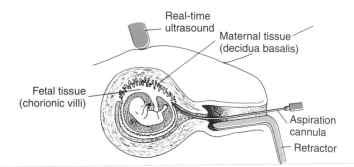

Figure 8-13
Chorionic villi sampling. Taking sample by transcervical method.
(From Bobak IM et al: *Maternity and gynecologic care: the nurse and the family,* ed 5, St. Louis, 1993, Mosby.)

12. Collagen vascular diseases
13. Older gravida (more than 35 years)
14. Chronic renal disease
15. Decreasing (or apparently absent) fetal movement
16. Severe maternal anemia
17. Discordant twins
18. Multiple gestation
19. High-risk antepartum patients (premature rupture of membranes, preterm labor, and bleeding)

Nonstress Test

Description

The basis for the NST to assess fetal well-being is that the normal fetus will produce characteristic heart rate patterns. Average baseline variability and acceleration of FHR in response to fetal movement are reassuring signs. The FHR pattern is assessed by external monitoring techniques without any stress or stimuli to the fetus.

When hypoxia, acidosis, or drugs depress the fetal central nervous system, there may be a reduction in baseline variability and absence of FHR acceleration with fetal movement. The patterns can also be produced by quiet fetal sleep states, and therefore it is sometimes necessary to monitor 20 to 30 minutes or more until the fetus is in a more active state or to palpate the abdomen or use vibroacoustic stimulation (VAS) to activate the resting fetus.

Contraindications

There are no contraindications to the NST.

Preparation and Procedure

An advantage of the NST over the CST is that it can be performed in an outpatient setting. Prepare the patient for the NST by taking a baseline blood pressure, then applying the external mode of monitoring with the patient in semi-Fowler's position and with a lateral tilt (Figure 8-14).

The observer identifies fetal movement on the chart paper as evidenced by spikes or momentary increases in uterine pressure. The new generation of EFMs are sensitive to fetal movements and mark their occurrence. If evidence of fetal movement is not apparent on the chart paper, the patient is asked to depress an event button when she perceives fetal movement. The "event" of fetal movement is

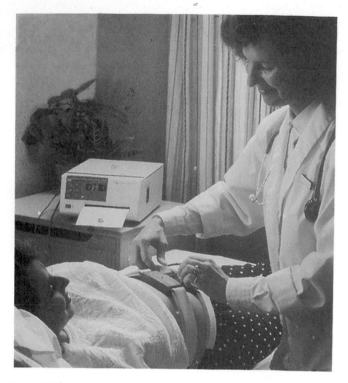

Figure 8-14
Antepartum monitoring.
(Courtesy Corometrics Medical Systems, Inc., Wallingford, Conn.)

then noted by a vertical line printed by the stylus on the uterine activity (UA) section of the monitor strip. Fetal monitors with Doppler fetal movement detection capability detect movements automatically and record them simultaneously with FHR and uterine activity. These monitors have been shown to detect gross fetal trunk movements with a very good correlation to such ultrasound-detected movements (Melendez, Rayburn, and Smith, 1992; Besinger and Johnson, 1989). This capability is important in that fetal movement is not always accurately perceived by the mother. In addition, this FHR-FMP (Fetal Movement Profile) employs two of the five parameters of the Biophysical Profile and its use may avoid the necessity of a contraction stress test (Stanco et al, 1993).

If necessary, fetal movement can be facilitated by palpation of the abdomen or VAS to activate the fetus. If indicated, maternal blood pressure may be monitored during and at the end of the procedure. The procedure usually lasts 20 minutes but may need to be extended if criteria for a reactive pattern have not been met. If the pattern is questionable or if decelerations occur, a biophysical profile (BPP) and/or CST may then be performed, or monitoring may be continued until interpretable data are obtained.

Interpretation

The following guidelines for evaluation of the NST are offered, although minor variations in criteria are successfully used by various institutions.

Reactive test (Figure 8-15)	Two or more FHR accelerations above baseline of at least 15 bpm lasting at least 15 seconds in a 20-minute period; baseline rate is within the normal range, and variability is average
Nonreactive test (Figure 8-16)	Absence of accelerations of FHR during the testing period
Inconclusive test	Less than one acceleration above baseline in a 20-minute period or one that is less than 15 bpm and lasts less than 15 seconds; variability less than 6 bpm or quality of FHR recording not adequate for interpretation

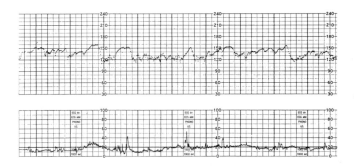

Figure 8-15
Reactive nonstress test (FHR acceleration with fetal movement).

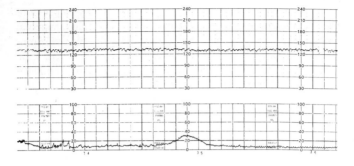

Figure 8-16
Nonreactive nonstress test (no FHR acceleration with fetal movement).

Clinical Significance and Management

The reactive test suggests that the fetus will be born in good condition if labor occurs in a few days. However, when the NST is used for primary fetal surveillance, it should be performed twice weekly in high-risk patients, especially those with postdate pregnancies and diabetes or IUGR. As long as twice-weekly NSTs remain reactive, most high-risk pregnancies are allowed to continue. The nonreactive test should be followed as soon as possible by a contraction stress test (CST). Patients with an inconclusive test may have the NST repeated in several hours, or may have a CST or biophysical profile (BPP), according to the clinical assessment of the physician.

Inasmuch as a nonreactive or inconclusive test can be caused by fetal sleep states, an attempt should be made to stimulate the fetus by manipulating the uterus or by stimulating the fetus with vibro-acoustic stimulation (VAS) and continuing to monitor the fetus for another 20- or 30-minute period.

Current trends reported in the literature are to combine NST with amniotic fluid index (AFI) readings of BPP in the fetal surveillance of high-risk pregnancies. Depending on gestational age or deliver-ability, the nonreactive test should be followed as soon as possible by a BPP and/or CST. Patients with an inconclusive test may have the NST repeated in several hours, or may have a BPP and/or CST, according to the clinical assessment of the physician.

Vibroacoustic Stimulation

Vibroacoustic stimulation (VAS) is another method of testing FHR response. The procedure is as follows:

1. Monitor the FHR and uterine activity until at least 10 minutes of interpretable data are obtained. If there are no spontaneous accelerations of FHR, then proceed to the next step.
2. Apply the artificial larynx or a fetal acoustic stimulation device firmly to the maternal abdomen over the fetal head.
3. Depress the button on the device for a single 1- to 2-second sound stimulation. (At the same time, it is preferable to depress the event marker, which will mark the uterine activity panel of the monitor strip.)
4. Observe and document the FHR response.
5. Repeat stimulus at 1-minute intervals up to three times if accelerations do not occur after the first acoustic stimulus.

Interpretation

Reactive Test: Two FHR accelerations of 15 bpm above baseline for 15 seconds in response to acoustic stimulation within 10 minutes
Nonreactive Test: Inability to fulfill the criterion for reactivity as described above within 10 minutes

Clinical Significance and Management

Management for the patient with a reactive test includes ongoing surveillance. Those with a nonreactive test should have a BPP and/or CST performed. Practice and literature differ in duration and number of repetitions of stimulation and criteria for describing reassuring and nonreassuring results. Some studies report fetal tachycardias that result from VAS, with heart rates that take up to 5 minutes or more to return to baseline. Some believe that when VAS is used to save time in performing an NST (not to wait for spontaneous fetal movements), sleep cycles may be disrupted. Normative data on potential effects of VAS are still being collected and analyzed and warrant caution when abnormal diagnoses are made based on this test alone (Gegor and Paine, 1992).

Contraction Stress Test

The basis for the CST is that a healthy fetus can withstand a decreased oxygen supply during the physiological stress of a contraction, whereas a compromised fetus will demonstrate late decelerations that are nonreassuring and indicative of uteroplacental insufficiency.

CSTs can be performed with endogenously produced oxytocin as stimulated by breast and nipple manipulation, or the test can be performed with an exogenous source of oxytocin administered by intravenous infusion.

Although the NST can be performed on any patient, the CST cannot. The potential for preterm labor precludes performing the test on patients with certain high-risk conditions and gestational ages.

The CST is contraindicated in the following situations:

1. Premature rupture of membranes
2. Placenta previa
3. Third-trimester bleeding
4. Previous classical cesarean section
5. Multiple gestation
6. Incompetent cervix
7. Hydramnios
8. History of preterm labor

The two types of CST are the nipple-stimulated contraction stress test and the oxytocin challenge test.

Nipple-Stimulated Contraction Stress Test

Procedure	Rationale
1. Assist the patient to a semi-Fowler's position with lateral tilt	1. To avoid supine hypotension
2. Place the tocotransducer where the least maternal tissue is in evidence, usually above the umbilicus	2. To ensure that the fundus is as close as possible to the pressure-sensing device
3. Place the ultrasound transducer on the maternal abdomen where the clearest fetal signal can be obtained	3. To ensure that the tracing is clear and interpretable

Procedure	Rationale
4. Monitor baseline FHR and uterine activity until 10 minutes of interpretable data are obtained (defer nipple stimulation if three spontaneous unstimulated contractions of more than 40 seconds duration occur within a 10-minute period)	4. To provide a basis for comparison (it may not be necessary to proceed with test if spontaneous contractions occur)
5. Instruct patient to brush palmar surface of the fingers over the nipple of one breast through her clothes; continue four cycles of 2 minutes on and 2 to 5 minutes off; stop when contraction begins and restimulate when contraction ends (if a 2-minute period has elapsed)	5. To stimulate oxytocin secretion into the circulation from the pituitary gland
a. If unsuccessful after four cycles, restimulate the breasts for 10 minutes, stopping when contraction begins and resuming when contraction ends	a. To maintain uterine contractions
b. If unsuccessful, begin bilateral continuous stimulation for 10 minutes, stopping when contraction begins and resuming when contraction ends	
6. Discontinue nipple stimulation when three or more spontaneous contractions lasting longer than 40 seconds occur in a 10-minute period and are palpable to the examiner. Discontinue the oxytocin anytime there is evidence of hyperstimulation, prolonged bradycardia, or consistent late decelerations;	6. To eliminate unnecessary stress

Procedure	Rationale
treat fetal distress in the same manner as during intrapartum monitoring; be prepared to administer terbutaline for tocolysis	
7. Interpret results and continue monitoring until uterine activity has returned to the prestimulation state	7. To ensure that the patient and fetus are restored to their prestress status

If nipple stimulation does not produce the desired uterine activity, an oxytocin-stimulated CST is indicated. Interpretation guidelines for contraction stress testing are described after the oxytocin challenge test (OCT).

Oxytocin Challenge Test

The oxytocin challenge test (OCT) is routinely performed in the inpatient setting because labor may be stimulated in some sensitive patients, particularly in those at term.

Procedure	Rationale
1. Assist patient into a semi-Fowler's position with lateral tilt	1. To avoid supine hypotension
2. Place the tocotransducer where the least maternal tissue is in evidence, usually above the umbilicus	2. To ensure that the fundus is as close as possible to the pressure-sensing button
3. Place the ultrasound transducer where the clearest fetal heart sound can be heard, usually below the umbilicus	3. To obtain a clear fetal signal
4. Monitor baseline FHR and uterine activity until 10 minutes of interpretable data are obtained before administration of oxytocin	4. To provide a basis for comparison
5. Check the patient's blood pressure and pulse every 10 to 15 minutes	5. To identify hypotension resulting from maternal position

Procedure	Rationale
6. If less than three spontaneous unstimulated contractions occur within a 10-minute period and if late decelerations do note occur with spontaneous contractions, oxytocin can be initiated	6. Oxytocin stimulation may not be necessary if adequate uterine activity is present; test may be discontinued if late decelerations occur with spontaneous contractions
7. Piggyback oxytocin into the primary IV line (with lactated Ringer's or other nonaqueous solution) near IV hub	7. May be necessary to stop oxytocin and rapidly infuse the primary IV in the event of uterine hyperstimulation or maternal hypotension
8. Administer oxytocin beginning with 0.5-2.0 mU/minute with a constant infusion pump per unit protocol	8. To ensure specific dosage of oxytocin
9. Increase the dosage of oxytocin infusion by 0.5-1.0 mU/minute at 15-minute intervals until the contraction frequency is three in 10 minutes of 40 to 60 seconds duration and contractions are palpable to the examiner	9. To ensure a safe rate of oxytocin increments; generally the dosage of oxytocin does not exceed 5 mU/minute, but occasional doses of up to 10 mU/minute may be necessary
10. Discontinue the oxytocin when three contractions have occurred within a 10-minute period of interpretable data	10. To provide an adequate stress from which an interpretation can be made
11. Discontinue the oxytocin any time there is evidence of hyperstimulation, prolonged bradycardia, or consistent late decelerations; treat fetal distress in the same manner as during intrapartum monitoring; be prepared to administer terbutaline for tocolysis	11. To prevent additional fetal distress; the principles for treating fetal distress apply during both antepartum and intrapartum monitoring
12. Continue to monitor until uterine activity and FHR return to baseline status	12. To ensure that the patient and fetus are restored to their prestress status

Interpretation

1. Negative test (Figure 8-17)	1. Three uterine contractions in a 10-minute period without late decelerations; there is usually average baseline variability and acceleration of FHR with fetal movement
2. Positive test (Figure 8-18)	2. Persistent late decelerations or late decelerations with more than half the contractions; may be associated with minimal or absent variability
3. Suspicious test	3. Late decelerations occurring with less than half the uterine contractions
4. Hyperstimulation	4. Contractions occurring more often than every 2 minutes or lasting longer than 90 seconds, or if there is apparent hypertonus associated with contractions; if no late decelerations occur with the preceding, the test is interpreted as negative; if late deceleration is observed during or after excessive uterine activity, the test is not interpretable and is classified as hyperstimulation because the stress is considered enough to exceed even normal uteroplacental reserve
5. Unsatisfactory	5. Quality of the recording is not sufficient to be sure that no late decelerations are present or where less than three uterine contractions have occurred in a 10-minute period; the test is not interpretable and cannot be used for clinical management

The CST is highly reliable when it is negative. False negatives are rare. On the other hand, false positives can occur if hyperstimulation patterns are unrecognized or if maternal position is supine, resulting in hypotension and late decelerations.

In contrast, when there is an absence of late decelerations in a patient in labor with a previous positive CST, it may be indicative of a correction of uteroplacental insufficiency in the interval between the test and labor and not a false positive CST.

Clinical Significance and Management

A negative CST is reassuring that the fetus is likely to survive labor should it occur within 1 week, as long as there is no change in sta-

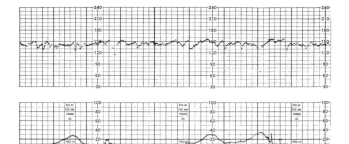

Figure 8-17
Negative contraction stress test (reassuring external tracing).

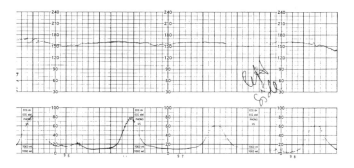

Figure 8-18
Positive contraction stress test (late deceleration with uterine contractions).

tus of either the mother or the fetus. This may permit a postponement of intervention until fetal lung maturity is achieved. As an indicator of fetoplacental respiratory reserve, the CST cannot prevent fetal death from obstetrical emergencies such as abruptio placentae and prolapsed cord. Preterm labor is not associated with a CST. If the fetus is less than 38 weeks gestation, labor almost never begins within 48 hours after the procedure.

Immediate retesting is required if there is a sudden change in maternal condition of the following: lupus flare, diabetes out of control, sickle cell crisis, worsening preeclampsia/pregnancy-induced hypertension, worsening renal disease, severe maternal dehydration, and an acute asthmatic episode.

The literature reports a false positive rate as high as 30% (Gegor and Paine, 1992). Therefore management of the patient with a positive CST is not clear cut. Fetal assessment utilizing other techniques such as BPP is indicated. In some cases, immediate termination of pregnancy may be warranted.

Home Uterine Activity Monitoring for Patients at Risk of Preterm Labor

Home uterine activity monitoring has been used in an attempt to prevent preterm births. This has been achieved with the utilization of a lightweight tocodynamometer designed for ambulatory home monitoring, data storage, and telephone transmission of uterine activity. Patients using this device have been given detailed instructions regarding the frequency of self-monitoring and asked to phone daily transmissions to a central monitoring unit. An obstetrical nurse interprets the data and then advises the patient as appropriate for the uterine activity noted on the transmission. The patient may be told to take additional tocolytic agents, increase hydration, empty the bladder, be remonitored, and then be referred to a primary care center for further evaluation (Stringer et al, 1994). Some visiting nursing or home health nursing agencies perform home monitoring in conjunction with a home visit. Thus the nurse is present during the monitoring and can perform further physical evaluation (palpation and vaginal examination) if warranted by the assessed uterine activity. Self-palpation by the patient is another method of monitoring uterine activity without a monitor but with daily telephone contact between the patient and a nurse.

However, to date prospective studies do not support the efficacy of home uterine activity monitoring. Data suggest that the time period during which contractions are detected either by home monitoring or self-palpation is limited to 12 to 24 hours before preterm birth (Iams, Johnson, and Parker, 1994) and this time frame may not be sufficient to allow for treatment before cervical changes occur that can lead to preterm birth. Daily provider-initiated telephone contact may be as effective as home uterine activity monitoring in a select group of women prospectively identified as at risk for preterm birth. Frequent provider contact, heightened patient awareness of the signs and symptoms of preterm birth, self-palpation, and home uterine activity monitoring are all only as effective as the timeliness or window of opportunity identified to delay the onset of labor. The controversy continues as to the overall effectiveness of these actions in the prevention of preterm births.

Care of the Monitored Patient

9

Use of EFM for antepartum and intrapartum patients is a standard of care for both low- and high-risk pregnancies. Also considered the standard of care is the use of EFM in high-risk pregnancies for nonstress testing (NST) and stress testing during the antepartum period. It is an expectation that nurses maintain adequate tracings and interpret baseline characteristics and periodic and nonperiodic changes. It is a standard of care for nurses to identify various patterns; document assessments, interpretations, and interventions; and notify appropriate people (e.g., obstetricians, neonatologists, and midwives) in a timely manner. Failure to do otherwise is practicing below the standard of practice and leaves nurses liable for their action or inaction.

One must keep in mind that the EFM, regardless of its level of sophistication, is only one tool used for fetal surveillance. A FHR tracing should never be the only assessment method used to determine fetal well-being. Other assessment data that must be interpreted concurrently with the tracing include subjective patient data, objective findings acquired from physical examination of the patient, laboratory data, and information obtained from ultrasound examination.

The care given to the continuously monitored patient in labor is the same care given to any patient during labor, with additional consideration to those factors that relate directly to the monitor. The most important item by far is a thorough explanation to the patient and her partner and support people about the monitor—how it is used, how it is applied, and what is being evaluated. Many patients are anxious about the status of the baby, concluding that something must be wrong that necessitates the monitor use. Some patients fear the machine itself and are distracted by its mechanical

noises and beeps. Others are afraid to move in bed for fear of dis-
lodging the leads and are concerned that the leads may harm the
baby.

The digital display of FHR is also frequently a source of anxiety.
Because the EFM cannot print out every heartbeat, sampling of
FHR is displayed and often very low or very high numbers are observed. Patients expressing concern over these numbers should be
told that variations in the displayed FHR are to be expected.

Often, the monitor is reassuring to the patient. An audible
"beep" of the fetal heart sounds can be reassuring that all is well
with the fetus. This sound often serves as encouragement to the patient, especially during active labor when some patients, over-
whelmed by their discomfort, lose sight of the imminent birth of
their baby. For those patients who feel discouraged about labor, it
is often reassuring to see evidence of uterine contractions. Visual-
izing contractions can also help the support person guide the laboring patient through the contraction by using breathing, focus,
and relaxation techniques.

There is no contraindication to showing the patient and her support person the monitor strip differentiating FHR from uterine activity. Even when this is not shown to them, they quickly identify
and contrast the FHR from the uterine activity (UA) panel without
much difficulty. Patients do observe changes in the monitoring pattern, such as those caused by fetal movement, and can be given appropriate explanations when decelerations or dips in the FHR occur. After all, in an emergency situation there are no real secrets
about the urgency of the situation.

Whether a patient is continuously monitored during labor, the
care and issues involving documentation are the same. The monitor
should not receive more attention than the patient (Figure 9-1). During the antepartum and intrapartum period, the OB nurse is responsible for two patients, maternal and fetal. This necessitates the use of
both maternal and fetal surveillance, which includes risk assessments determined through history taking, physical examination, and
biochemical and biophysical testing. Laboring patients are monitored for progress of labor, maternal well-being, pain management,
psychosocial evaluation, and cultural needs. Intrapartum surveillance evaluates fetal tolerance of labor and determines fetal well-
being. Guidelines for care are described in the following quick-ref-
erence outline.

Care of the Monitored Patient
Observations

Patient's position
Patient's comfort
Respiratory rate and pattern
Temperature
Blood pressure
Voiding pattern
Uterine contraction pattern: frequency, duration, intensity, resting tone
Fetal heart rate, baseline rate, variability, periodic and nonperiodic changes

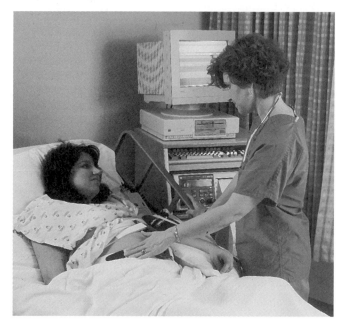

Figure 9-1
The nurse manages the care of the monitored patient, ensuring that the monitor does not receive more attention than the patient.
(Courtesy Corometrics Medical Systems, Inc., Wallingford, Conn.)

Placement and functioning of external transducers (tocotransducer, ultrasound transducer) and internal devices (spiral electrode, intrauterine pressure catheter)

Adjustment and repositioning of equipment

Cervical effacement and dilatation

Fetal presentation and position

Status of membranes

Color and amount of amniotic fluid

Ongoing Care

Verify clock time/calendar date on monitor; verify monitor to room clock and computer if using electronic documentation

Test monitor on initiation and as needed (Table 9-1)

Position patient comfortably

Encourage lateral position if bed is flat (modify this if patient is in semi-Fowler's position) to prevent supine hypotension syndrome

Chart all nursing and patient care activities on monitor strip

During the first stage of labor:

Document FHR q15 to 30 min (in low-risk patients)

When risk factors are present, document FHR q15 min when intermittent auscultation is used; if the patient is electronically monitored, the strip chart should be evaluated q15 to 30 min and initialed to verify this

During the second stage of labor

Evaluate and record the FHR q5 min when auscultation is used in patients with risk factors

Evaluate the FHR strip chart on electronically monitored patients with risk factors q5 min

In low-risk patients the FHR should be documented q15 min (if auscultated) or the strip chart reviewed, evaluated, and initialed for patients who are electronically monitored

Document FHR immediately after membranes rupture and again in 5 min

External Monitoring

Ultrasound Transducer

(Monitors FHR with high-frequency sound waves)

Use *Leopold's maneuvers* to assist in determining fetal lie to clearly locate FHR

Table 9-1   Fetal monitoring equipment checklist

Name: _____ Date: _____	Evaluator: _____		
Items To Be Checked	Yes	No	Remarks
Preparation of Monitor 1. Is the paper inserted correctly? 2. Are the transducer cables plugged securely into the appropriate outlet?			
Ultrasound Transducer 1. Has transmission gel been applied to the transducer? 2. Was the FHR tested and noted on the monitor strip? 3. Does an audible beep or signal light flash with each heartbeat? 4. Is the strap secure and snug?			
Tocotransducer 1. Is the tocotransducer firmly strapped where the least maternal tissue is in evidence? 2. Has it been applied without gel or paste? 3. Was the penset knob adjusted between the 10 and 20 mm marks and noted on chart paper? 4. Was this setting done between contractions? 5. Is the strap secure and snug?			
Spiral Electrode 1. Are the wires attached firmly to the leg plate? 2. Is the spiral electrode attached to the presenting part of the fetus? 3. Is the inner surface of the leg plate covered with electrode paste (if necessary)? 4. Is the leg plate properly secured to the patient's thigh?			

Continued

Table 9-1 Fetal monitoring equipment checklist—cont'd

Name: _____	Evaluator: _____		
Date: _____			
Items To Be Checked	Yes	No	Remarks
Internal Catheter			
1. Is the length line on the catheter visible at the introitus?			
2. Is it noted on the chart paper that a calibration was done?			
3. Has the catheter been properly zeroed according to institution policy and procedure?			
4. Is the catheter properly secured to patient?			
5. Is baseline resting tone of uterus documented?			

Tap transducer with finger before use to ensure sound transmission

Apply ultrasound transmission gel to maternal abdomen

Clean abdomen and transducer and reapply gel prn

Massage reddened skin areas and reposition belt prn

Auscultate FHR with Doppler or fetoscope if in doubt as to the validity of monitor strip and compare with maternal pulse

Position and reposition transducer as needed to ensure clear interpretable FHR data; massage reddened areas prn

Tocotransducer

(Monitors uterine activity via a pressure-sensing device placed on the maternal abdomen) (Figure 9-2)

Palpate abdomen and position and reposition tocotransducer as needed on the fundus where the least maternal tissue is in evidence

Maintain snug abdominal strap

Adjust penset *between* contractions to print between 10 and 20 mm Hg on the monitor strip

Palpate fundus every 30 to 60 minutes to gauge strength of contraction; only frequency and duration of contractions can be assessed with tocotransducer

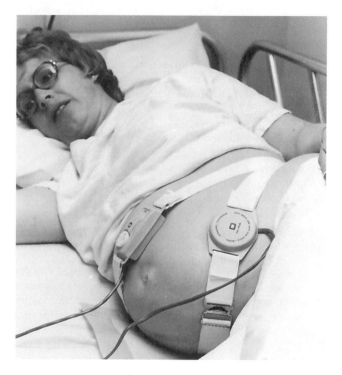

Figure 9-2
Externally monitored patient in side-lying position.

Do not assess patient's need for analgesia based on uterine activity displayed on strip; listen to patient's subjective viewpoint regarding contraction intensity, resting tone, and level of pain

Reposition belt and transducer q2 hr and prn and massage reddened skin areas prn; document and avoid areas of skin breakdown

Internal Monitoring
Spiral Electrode

(Obtains fetal ECG from presenting part and converts to FHR)
Ensure that color-coded wires are appropriately attached to push post on leg plate if indicated

Apply electrode paste to leg plate prn

Observe FHR panel of strip chart for long- and short-term variability

Turn electrode counterclockwise to remove; *never* pull straight out from presenting part

Administer perineal care after voiding and prn

Intrauterine Catheter

(Catheter internally monitors intrauterine pressure)

Ensure that length line on catheter is visible at introitus

For fluid-filled catheters, turn stopcock off to patient, release pressure valve of strain gauge, flush strain gauge, remove syringe, and set printer to 0 line on monitor paper; test further as needed, according to manufacturer's instructions

Check proper functioning by tapping catheter, asking patient to cough, or applying fundal pressure; observe appropriate inflection on monitor strip

The newest intrauterine pressure catheters are equipped with dual lumens, internal transducers, and amnioports. One lumen is designated as the internal transducer. The second lumen is designated for amnioinfusion. Some may have precalibrated computer chips located in the tip and require no fluid. Some have the capacity to be rezeroed while still in place inside the patient

Keep catheter secured to patient's leg to prevent dislodgment

Patient Teaching

Ensure that the patient and her support person(s) know and understand that the:

Use of the monitor does not imply fetal jeopardy

Fetal status via FHR can be continuously assessed even during contractions

Lower panel on the strip chart shows uterine activity and that the upper panel shows FHR

Prepared childbirth techniques can be implemented without difficulty

Effleurage performed during external monitoring can be done on the sides of the abdomen or upper thighs

Breathing patterns based on timing and intensity of contraction can be enhanced by observation of the uterine activity panel of the strip chart for onset of contractions

    Note peak of contraction; knowing that contraction will not
       get stronger and is half over is usually helpful
    Note diminishing intensity
    Coordinate with appropriate breathing and relaxation techniques
  Use of internal mode of monitoring does not restrict patient
    movement
  Use of external mode of monitoring usually requires patient co-
    operation in positioning and movement

Documentation

The adage "if it was not documented, then it was not done" clearly ap-
plies to fetal monitoring and care of the patient in labor, especially
when this information may be reviewed months or years later in legal
action. It is imperative to have excellent records (Figure 9-3). Infor-

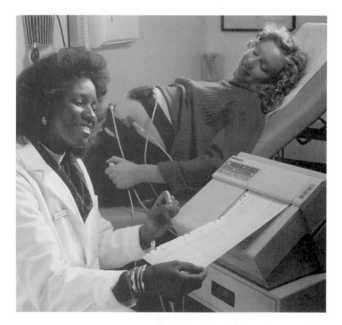

Figure 9-3
Documentation is easily achieved by handwriting notes
directly on the strip chart in this slant top monitor.
(Courtesy Hewlett-Packard, Böblingen, Germany.)

mation that should be included on the monitor strip, standard chart, or electronic record beginning, during, and after monitoring follows:

1. Beginning of monitoring
   a. Patient's name and age
   b. Identification number
   c. Date
   d. Physician's name
   e. Time the monitor was attached and mode
   f. Testing/calibration
   g. Gravida _____ Para _____
   h. Expected date of confinement (EDC)
   i. Monitor code number
   j. High-risk factors (e.g., pregnancy-induced hypertension, diabetes)
   k. Membranes intact or ruptured
   l. Gestational age
   m. Dilatation and station

2. During the course of monitoring
   a. Maternal position and repositioning in bed
   b. Vaginal examination and results
   c. Analgesia or anesthesia
   d. Medication given
   e. BP, T, P, and R
   f. Voidings
   g. O$_2$ given
   h. Emesis
   i. Pushing
   j. Fetal movement
   k. Any change in mode of monitoring
   l. Adjustments of equipment
      (1) Relocation of transducers
      (2) Type and adjustment of catheter
      (3) Replacement of electrode
      (4) Replacement or removal of catheter
   m. All identification and interventions for nonreassuring FHR patterns

   If you know what it is—name it
   If the pattern is unknown—describe it
   If the pattern is indescribable—draw it

   n. Document to parameters for first and second stages of labor as listed on p. 170.

This ensures that someone has assessed the patient and FHR on a regular basis and ensures that a nonreassuring pattern is observed and subsequently treated.

This is important for retrospective audit and teaching purposes and is of the utmost importance in identifying the cause of a specific FHR response to nursing or medical action.

3. On completion of monitoring and delivery, the nurse should make the following summary notations at the end of the chart paper:
   a. Delivery date and time
   b. Type of delivery
   c. Anesthesia
   d. Sex and weight of the infant
   e. Presentation
   f. Both 1- and 5-minute Apgar scores
   g. Complications
   h. Presence or absence of meconium
   i. Cord blood pH, if done

The monitor strip then presents a complete picture of the patient's labor.

Pattern Interpretation

Interpretation of the FHR pattern and uterine activity should be done in a thorough, systematic fashion. The baseline FHR should be identified as being within the normal fetal heart range, tachycardia, or bradycardia. The degree of baseline variability should be assessed, noting the presence or absence of short- and long-term variability. Periodic changes should be noted as spontaneous or periodic accelerations of FHR and early, late, or variable decelerations. Uterine activity should be assessed by the frequency and duration of contractions, and if the patient is monitored internally, the intensity and resting tone of the uterus in millimeters of mercury pressure is identified. A tool for assessment of the fetal monitor strip chart is offered in Table 9-2 and can be used when monitoring is in progress or after delivery for teaching or quality improvement purposes.

The significance of appropriate use of equipment and assessment of the FHR monitor strip cannot be overemphasized. Individuals caring for patients sometimes have the opportunity to review their documentation during legal proceedings. The prudent caretaker will ensure that all equipment is appropriately used and that patient care activities, including assessment and interventions, are appropriate and documented in a clear, concise, and objective manner.

Table 9-2   Fetal heart rate assessment checklist

Patient's Name _____ Date/Time _____

1. What is the baseline fetal heart rate (FHR)?
   _____ Beats per minute (bpm)
   Check one of the following as observed on the monitor strip:
   _____ Average baseline FHR (120 to 160 bpm)
   _____ Tachycardia (>120 bpm or >30 bpm from normal/previous baseline)
   _____ Bradycardia (<120 bpm or <30 bpm from normal/previous baseline)
2. What is the baseline variability?
   _____ Average short-term variability (6 to 10 bpm)
   _____ Average long-term variability (3 to 5 cycles per minute)
   _____ Minimal variability
   _____ Absence of variability
   _____ Marked variability
3. Are there any periodic changes in FHR?
   _____ Accelerations with fetal movement
   _____ Repetitive accelerations with each contraction
   _____ Early decelerations (head compression)
   _____ Late decelerations (uteroplacental insufficiency)
   Variable decelerations (cord compression)
   _____ Mild
   _____ Moderate
   _____ Severe
4. What does the uterine activity panel show?
   _____ Frequency (onset to onset of UC or peak to peak)
   _____ Duration (beginning to end)
   _____ Intensity (in mm Hg only with intrauterine catheter)
   _____ Resting time at least 30 seconds
   _____ Resting tone (<15 mm Hg pressure)
COMMENTS: _____

PANEL NUMBER	WHAT CAN BE OR SHOULD HAVE BEEN DONE

Professional Issues

10

Legal Aspects

The nurse is legally responsible for performing fetal monitoring according to the established standard of care as defined by the nurse's employer and the nurse's professional education, medical practice, professional organizations, and the local state nurse practice act. Observations, evaluation, and intervention for the patient's symptoms, progress, and reactions are the nurse's responsibility within legally sanctioned confines. The nurse who develops expertise in monitoring and pattern recognition is held responsible for this expertise.

Increasing concern for competency in fetal monitoring has stimulated discussion and emphasized a trend toward the need for validating that competency, such as by a written certification examination. Electronic fetal monitoring is but one method of fetal assessment and cannot conceptually, or practically, be separated from other clinical assessment techniques or from the normal, high risk, physiological, and pathophysiological processes that may occur during the antepartum and intrapartum periods.

Electronic fetal monitoring is one part of a group of competencies based on a continuum of knowledge that the nurse must possess to care for antepartum and intrapartum patients. With the intent of promoting competency in clinical nursing practice, the Association of Women's Health, Obstetric, and Neonatal Nurses (AWHONN, formerly NAACOG) has developed *Electronic Fetal Monitoring: Nursing Practice Competencies and Educational Guidelines.* The guidelines describe minimal educational preparation to achieve competency in electronic fetal monitoring and are an excellent resource for the practicing nurse, nurse manager, or administrator, as well as the nursing educator (see Appendix G).

These AWHONN guidelines offer a way to categorize nursing responsibilities in electronic fetal monitoring. From closed claim and expert review, it is apparent that nursing responsibility, and therefore liability, seems to fall into the following categories: obtaining the data, interpretation of the data, nursing intervention based on the data, notification of the appropriate practitioner, and documentation.

Obtaining the Data

Whether electronic fetal monitoring is required for a particular patient is a clinical decision that is made prospectively using data available to the practitioner at the time of the decision. This decision is also based on the policies, procedures, and standards of practice in a given institution. Although the "standard of care" may not **require** the use of an electronic fetal monitor, it is incumbent upon the nurse to use it properly once it is placed into use.

Hours of "chicken scratching" do not show that any standard of care has been met simply because an electronic fetal monitor was on the patient. The charge to the perinatal nurse is to obtain and maintain an adequate tracing of the fetal heart and uterine contractions (NAACOG, 1991). The nurse must also be able to identify technically inadequate tracings and take appropriate corrective action (AAP/ACOG, 1992). Thirty minutes is generally the acceptable limit for an electronic fetal monitor tracing that is not interpretable. If the nurse is unable to continuously monitor the fetal heart, the nurse should document the attempts to adjust the monitor and note the fetal heart rate per auscultation until an interpretable tracing can be obtained. If all efforts prove unsuccessful, the nurse should notify the patient's primary care provider so that alternative methods of assessing the fetal heart rate may be explored.

Care must also be taken to obtain an adequate uterine contraction tracing. In one claim that resulted in a $2.2 million settlement, only the Doppler transducer was applied, with no tocotransducer used for uterine contraction monitoring. The fact that the nurses failed to use the tocotransducer resulted in an inability to evaluate the nature of decelerations that became evident on the monitor strip. A prudent nurse would have taken steps to obtain a complete strip in order to appropriately evaluate fetal well-being.

Before the widespread use of Labor/Delivery/Recovery rooms (LDRs) there was a spate of cases where electronic fetal monitoring had been discontinued too soon. These involved patients who had been electronically monitored throughout their labors, but upon being transferred to the traditional "delivery room" had their electronic monitors discontinued and not brought over to the delivery room for continued monitoring. The AAP/ACOG guidelines are quite clear that the standard of practice for monitoring low-risk patients in the second stage of labor is to evaluate—by either auscultation or electronic fetal monitor—and record the fetal heart rate at least every 15 minutes. When risk factors are present, the fetal heart rate should be evaluated and recorded at least every 5 minutes when auscultation is used and should be evaluated at least every 5 minutes when electronic fetal monitoring is used. It is recommended that facilities develop a policy to cover such situations. The absence of any documentation whatsoever of fetal heart rate monitoring, either by auscultation or electronic means, makes a case very difficult, if not impossible, to defend against charges of nursing negligence.

Interpretation of Data

In a landmark 1981 California case a verdict was returned in favor of a 3½-year-old child who was severely brain damaged since birth. The hospital was found totally liable, and the physician was exonerated. The physician attached the fetal monitor and went into his office, as everything on the monitor strip appeared to be normal. Within a short period of time, however, there appeared profound and persistent late decelerations. The nurse who was assigned to care for the patient had no education or training in electronic fetal monitoring and failed to interpret the presence of fetal distress on the monitor. The fetal monitor continued to display marked heart rate abnormalities up to the time that the nurse called the physician to come and deliver the baby when the patient was fully dilated. Although the physician delivered the baby as expeditiously as possible, the baby was severely depressed at birth and suffered profound brain damage. The nurse's deposition was particularly effective in proving that the nurse knew next to nothing about fetal monitor interpretation. Experts testified that a nurse working in Labor and Delivery should be able to interpret the information provided by a fetal monitor. The jury determined that the hospital had both indirect and direct liability in this case. The hospital was vicariously, or indirectly, liable for the nurse's failure to interpret the monitor strip accurately and directly liable for placing an incompetent nurse in Labor and Delivery (Rubsamen, 1993).

The AWHONN core competencies state that the nurse should be able to "identify baseline fetal heart rate and rhythm, variability, and the presence of periodic and nonperiodic changes," as well as be able to "determine if findings are reassuring or nonreassuring and implement appropriate nursing interventions" (NAACOG, 1991). It is also established law that nurses owe a duty to the patient to possess skills appropriate to their nursing function and that they must use **reasonable** care in the exercise of those skills. These statements should make it clear that the Labor and Delivery nurse should be able to interpret fetal monitor tracings and treat fetal distress with appropriate nursing intervention. As Dr. Barry Schifrin stated so succinctly: "To utilize the fetal monitor without the capacity to interpret the tracing is negligent" (Schifrin et al, 1985).

Nursing Intervention Based on the Data

Again, the AWHONN competencies state that the nurse will "determine if findings are reassuring or nonreassuring and implement appropriate nursing interventions." Such interventions include the accepted nursing interventions of position change(s); oxygen administration; discontinuation of oxytocin; possible vaginal examination; and, often, the obtaining of further data.

Documentation of nursing intervention should include the time and type of interventions instituted, **what the patient(s) response** was to the intervention, and each time that the physician or primary caregiver was notified. Documentation of the patient response to the intervention is crucial in the medical record, both for documenting either resolution or a continuation of the findings and for substantiating the rationale for the plan of action.

A problem of nursing intervention—or lack of intervention—often seen on claim and expert review is that all of the above nursing interventions were instituted except that of the discontinuation of oxytocin. Such a finding in the face of fetal distress is almost always indefensible. If there is frank or suspected fetal distress, the oxytocin **must be discontinued** until there is some resolution to the problem. Virtually all nursing policies state that oxytocin should be discontinued in the face of fetal distress. Such policies usually spell out clearly that the above nursing interventions are to be instituted at the nurse's discretion. Nurses are cautioned to know what their policies say, to adhere to them, and to review and update such policies on a regular basis for appropriateness, clarity, consistency, and feasibility.

Notification of the Appropriate Practitioner

After identification of a nonreassuring pattern, the nurse's responsibility does not cease with nursing intervention alone.

The NAACOG Position Statement on "Nursing Responsibilities in Implementing Intrapartum FHR Monitoring" (1992) (Appendix F) states that after the nurse has identified a nonreassuring pattern and instituted and documented appropriate nursing interventions, he or she is then responsible for notifying the physician or certified nurse-midwife. Once the physician or other practitioner has been notified of a nonreassuring pattern, the nurse can expect that person to respond. An institutional policy should be established for the nurse to follow should the physician/practitioner be unable to respond in a timely fashion. Should the physician be unfamiliar with monitoring, or have differences in interpretation, the nurse must follow hospital protocol for resolving the conflict.

A common scenario often put forth is that of the nurse who reports fetal distress from observed findings on a FHR tracing. The physician, not at the bedside, disputes the nurse's interpretation. What subsequent steps should the nurse take?

It is important to remember that when a physician and nurse disagree, both have an obligation to the patient(s) to discuss and resolve the issue. In the "real world" of the clinical setting, this must be done quickly to facilitate appropriate treatment. The most appropriate way to resolve differences of opinion are usually contained in the facility's "chain of command" policy (Figure 10-1). Regardless, the staff nurse is often in a better position to speak with the physician about the matter if the nurse has reviewed the concerns with the charge nurse or another nurse recognized as a knowledgeable source. Such conversations should be documented, as they constitute a "nursing consultation" and can be very valuable from a defense point. Nurses do consultations all the time but rarely document them, unlike their medical colleagues who carefully record all consultations.

If, after discussion of the issue, the physician and nurse cannot resolve their differences and the nurse feels that she cannot carry out the resulting order, the dilemma should be presented to the

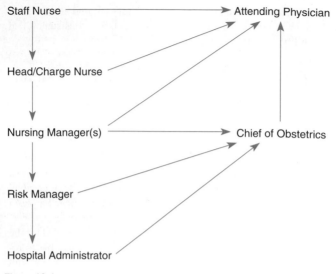

Figure 10-1
Sample chain-of-command for resolution of conflicts in
judgment between nurse(s) and attending physician.

charge nurse or supervisor. Generally, the next step is that the supervisor takes the issue to the Chief of Obstetrics. This lengthy
"chain of command" approach is only appropriate when there is sufficient time available. An accelerated approach must be instituted if
there is an emergent situation. The nurse must not waste time on the
more passive-aggressive approach of "assumptions," as in "I assumed the physician was coming"; "I assumed the physician knew
I needed him there right away"; and the ever-puzzling "I assumed
the physician knew what I meant."

Nursing documentation should reflect that the physician was
made aware of the FHR pattern and the time or times that the physician was notified.

Almost 30 years ago a California appellate decision, *Goff v. Doctors' Hospital* (1958), established the rule that a nurse has an independent professional duty to a patient. If it is within the nurse's professional competence to recognize that the doctor is neglecting the

patient, and the patient may suffer because of it, that nurse has an obligation to use the chain of command to remedy the situation. The legal obligation of the nurse to utilize the facility's chain of command policy has been made very clear over the last few decades and has done much to do away with the antiquated legal theory of "Captain of the Ship."

Documentation

The importance of documentation on the patient's medical record cannot be overemphasized. Adherence to standards of practice is essential, and appropriate assessment, intervention, and evaluation should be clearly documented. The practitioner should anticipate how the patient's record may be analyzed by others years after a delivery, as occurs during the litigation process. The general assumption is that what is not written did not occur, and the concept of what the reasonable, prudent nurse would do in the same situation takes on a new meaning to those who become involved in medical or nursing malpractice.

The patient's medical record should include baseline information such as the time that the fetal monitor was applied and the mode of monitoring being utilized. Specific FHR information should include the baseline fetal heart rate, an estimation of baseline variability whenever possible, and the presence and type of periodic patterns. Often overlooked, but equally important, are notations concerning baseline uterine resting tone and the presence, frequency, and duration of uterine contractions. Intensity of uterine contractions should be noted whenever an intrauterine pressure catheter is used.

It is appropriate to use the descriptive names that have been given to FHR patterns (e.g., accelerations and early, late, and variable decelerations) in written chart documentation and verbal communication. The use of narrative description is indicated when the monitor tracing does not fit the established criteria for the usual descriptive names. Nurses are cautioned against the use of terms such as "fetal distress," "fetal hypoxia," or "uteroplacental insufficiency" in their charting because these terms are **medical** diagnoses, and there are no consensus definitions for these terms. Charting the patterns' descriptive names, or the "reassuring" or "nonreassuring" characteristics of the patterns is of greater benefit.

If the findings on the monitor strip are nonreassuring, the nurse must embark on some course of remedial action and document those interventions and the time, or times, that the physician was notified of the pattern. Intervention notations should include the following:

- Time and type of nursing intervention initiated
- Patient response to the intervention
- The time(s) of physician notification and a summary of facts given to the physician. For example: "0535—Dr. Jones notified of the presence of late decelerations, which responded favorably to oxygen administration and position change"
- Any changes in the medical or nursing plan

Nurses should avoid the use of empty and meaningless charting phrases such as "physician notified of patient's condition." The chart should explain of what the physician was specifically notified. Such descriptive notes are invaluable should a problem arise years after the event. The following California case (Orimi, 1985) concerning perinatal brain damage illustrates this point all too clearly. The nurse had charted "Some decelerations noted; doctor advised of patient's condition." Questions arose during the discovery phase of litigation concerning the following: did the nurse telephone the obstetrician? (He did not recall speaking to her.) If she did call, what did she say? At the time of her deposition and testimony, she could not remember what she had or had not said to the obstetrician. The physician stated that had he only known of the decelerations, he would have gone immediately to the hospital to evaluate the patient. The jury accepted the physician's statement and the assertion by him that the nurse had provided too little information. The outcome of the trial was that the hospital was solely liable for damages totaling $5.8 million.

The overall goal of narrative medical record charting is to be accurate, objective, and free from editorial commentary, potentially damaging and biased comments, and "finger pointing." The medical record should never be used as the "battleground" but rather the means by which the health care professional can provide a clear, detailed, and objective account of the events as they occurred.

What goes in the patient's medical record and what goes on the strip chart? Do nurses have to chart everything in both places? These questions arise from valid concerns about nurses having to chart the same or similar information on multiple chart forms. The goal should be to make charting time efficient without sacrificing accuracy and completeness. The fetal monitor strip can be viewed as a convenient bedside flow sheet on which to record all patient- or provider-initiated activities related to patient care. Examples of these activities would include the following:

- Maternal status data, such as vital signs, activity or position changes, vaginal exam findings, or status of membranes
- Medications, including route, dosage, and time; medications may include analgesia or anesthesia, oxytocin, or tocolytics
- Nursing interventions, such as position changes, oxygen administration, discontinuation of oxytocin, vaginal exam findings, or hydration
- Delivery information, such as time and type of delivery, and baby information including sex, Apgar scores, weight, and any neonatal findings

When reviewing strip charts, it is disturbing to see hours of monitor tracing with no entries whatsoever on the strip. Such a tracing may suggest that no one observed that patient for the entire time, which is, fortunately, rarely the case. Often, the nurse may have observed and even assessed the patient, then determined that no further nursing action was necessary at the time. Nurses should be encouraged to chart at least the time and their initials on the strip chart whenever they are at a patient's bedside. A policy should be established at each facility as to how often the strip chart should be initialed when no scheduled patient care activities are taking place so as to document the physical presence or observation of the caregiver.

A properly documented strip chart should be able to stand alone with the information contained on it. However, the medical record should also be able to stand alone, because strip charts can and do disappear. The hospital medical records department is responsible for protecting hospital records from loss, defacement, tampering, and access by unauthorized individuals. Ideally, the monitor strips should be kept with the maternal medical record. Because of the bulkiness of electronic fetal monitor tracings, they are sometimes stored separately. If that is the case, they must be retrievable. Microfilm may be preferred for improved retention of tracings and ease of storage. Direct storage onto optical disk storage systems is probably optimal for storage, retention, and retrieval. Physicians, nurses, and administrators should be aware of their particular state's statutory regulations concerning the admissibility of computer-generated medical records in case of litigation. Care should be taken not to destroy the original hard copy of the monitor strip until this can be ascertained.

Claims experience has shown that if the fetal monitor tracings or any portion of them are missing, the claim has become virtually indefensible. Each year hospitals (or their liability insurance carriers) pay hundreds of thousands of dollars in settlements where the case may have been otherwise entirely defensible. The issue is one of economics, as well as liability.

As with any medical procedure, the patient has the right to refuse consent to be monitored. If a patient refuses the use of electronic fetal monitoring, the medical record should reflect that a thorough explanation of the reasons for EFM and its benefits has taken place. The explanation of risks, benefits, alternatives, and the risks of refusing a given procedure are all part of the informed consent process, which remains the nondelegable duty of the physician. Therefore the nurse must be certain that the physician is notified if a patient refuses monitoring. The medical record must then note that the patient understands the explanation that she has been given. If new risk factors develop, the patient should be given an explanation of the new indications and the explanation should be documented again. The record must reflect that a truly informed consent—or refusal—has taken place. As the patient advocate, it is the duty of the nurse to ascertain whether that process has taken place, and to notify the physician to remedy the situation if it has not.

The goal of fetal monitoring is to prevent or minimize potential fetal and maternal risk or injury. Adequate electronic fetal monitoring documentation facilitates assessment of maternal and fetal responses to nursing intervention, medication, and stresses such as uterine contractions. As with any documentation, it needs to be factual, objective, and timely. Careful documentation is essential to accurately reflect the quality of the care provided. Its importance has taken on greater significance because of the current malpractice environment.

Appendix A

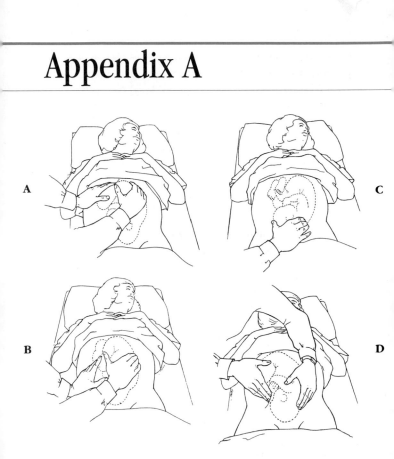

A-1
Leopold's maneuvers.

Leopold's Maneuvers and Determination of the Points of Maximum Intensity of the Fetal Heart Rate

Leopold's Maneuvers

Wash hands.

Ask woman to empty bladder.

Position woman supine with one pillow under her head and with her knees slightly flexed.

Place small rolled towel under woman's right hip to displace uterus to left off major blood vessels (avoids supine hypotensive syndrome).

If right-handed, stand on woman's right, facing her:

1. Identify fetal part that occupies the fundus. The head feels round, firm, freely movable, and palpable by ballottement; the breech feels less regular and softer (identifies fetal lie [vertical or horizontal] and presentation [vertex or breech]; Figure A-1, *A)*

2. Using palmar surface of one hand, locate and palpate the smooth convex contour of the fetal back and the irregularities that identify the small parts (feet, hands, elbows). This assists in identifying fetal presentation (Figure A-1, *B)*

3. With the right hand, determine which fetal part is presenting over the inlet to the true pelvis. Gently grasp the lower pole of the uterus between the thumb and fingers, pressing in slightly (Figure A-1, *C)*. If the head is presenting and not engaged, determine the attitude of the head.

4. Turn to face the woman's feet. Using two hands, outline the fetal head (Figure A-1, *D)* with palmar surface of fingertips.

When presenting part has descended deeply, only a small portion of it may be outlined.

Palpation of cephalic prominence assists in identifying attitude of head.

If the cephalic prominence is found on the same side as the small parts, the head must be flexed, and the vertex is presenting. If the cephalic prominence is on the same side as the back, the presenting head is extended.

From Bobak IM et al: Maternity nursing, ed 4, St. Louis, 1995, Mosby.

Leopold's Maneuvers and Determination of the Points of Maximum Intensity of the Fetal Heart Rate—cont'd

Determination of PMI of FHR:

Wash hands.

Perform Leopold's maneuvers.

Auscultate FHR.

Chart fetal presentation, position, and lie; whether presenting part is flexed or extended, engaged or free floating. Use hospital's protocol for charting (e.g., "Vtx, LOA, floating").

Chart PMI of FHR using a two-line figure to indicate the four quadrants of the maternal abdomen, right upper quadrant (RUQ), left upper quadrant (LUQ), left lower quadrant (LLQ), and right lower quadrant (RLQ):

RUQ	LUQ
RLQ	LLQ

The umbilicus is the point where the lines cross. The PMI for the fetus in vertex presentation, in general flexion with the back on the mother's right side, commonly is found in the mother's right lower quadrant and is recorded with an "x" or with the FHR as follows:

or

x | 140 |

Appendix B

Protocols for the Initiation of Labor: Cervical Ripening, Amniotomy, and Oxytocin Augmentation/Induction

Cervical Ripening

Cervical ripening changes the consistency of the uterus, making it softer and more distensible. This can be achieved by mechanical and chemical methods including stripping of the membranes, use of hygroscopic dilators, and the application of prostaglandin E_2 gel. Cervical ripening is desirable whenever induction of labor is indicated, the cervix is not favorable for induction, and there are no contraindications to the use of cervical ripening agents.

Stripping of the Membranes

Stripping of the membranes involves the digital separation of the membranes from the lower uterine segment. This is achieved through a vaginal examination, often with simultaneous pressure on the fundus of the uterus to ensure application of the vertex on the cervix.

The effects of membrane stripping are inconsistent and more likely to be effective with a higher Bishop score.

Possible complications

Bleeding from low-implanted placenta
Infection
Rupture of membranes

Hygroscopic Dilators

Synthetic hygroscopic dilators and laminaria tents (seaweed stems) placed into the endocervix absorb fluid, expand, and cause a dilator effect on the cervix. A number of dilators can be inserted under direct visualization and are held in place with povidone-iodine saturated gauze sponges.

Prostaglandin Gel

Local application of prostaglandin E_2 gel (PGE_2) is the most widely used cervical ripening agent. Prostaglandin E_2 gel placed onto the vagina or the cervical canal ripens the cervix. It should be administered only to patients for whom induction of labor is indicated.

Usual dosage

1. 0.5 mg when instilled in the endocervix
2. 2-3 mg when gel is placed intravaginally

Prostaglandin gel in a dosage of 0.5 mg has been commercially available since 1993. It is packaged in a pre-filled syringe. A catheter with a 10 or 20 mm tip is attached to the syringe to place the gel into the endocervix. The catheter is shielded to avoid application.

Guidelines for the use of prostaglandin gel

May be used up to 3 times, 6 hours apart

Should be applied by an appropriately credentialed health care provider.

Caution should be exercised when using in patients with history of asthma; glaucoma; or pulmonary, hepatic, or renal disease.

Use only in hospital setting when a physician who has delivery privileges to perform a cesarean delivery is readily available.

Patient should be instructed to remain supine for 15 to 30 minutes to minimize leakage of gel.

Store, warm, and prepare prostaglandin gel per supplier's instructions.

Monitor patient for uterine hyperstimulation and fetal heart rate changes by palpation and auscultation or continuous electronic fetal heart rate monitoring for 2 hours.

If hyperstimulation occurs, turn patient to lateral position, administer oxygen, and consider the use of a tocolytic agent.

If oxytocin is required, it should be started 6 to 12 hours following the last gel application.

Contraindications to prostaglandin gel

Patients in whom oxytocin is generally contraindicated

Patients with previous cesarean section with a classical incision or major uterine surgery

Patients with hypersensitivity to prostaglandins or constituents of the gel

Low-Dose Oxytocin Infusion

Oxytocin is considered a poor ripening agent; however, low-dose oxytocin administration may ripen the cervix.

Dosage

Starting dose:	0.5 milliunits per minute
Increase dose:	1 milliunit per hour
Maximum dose:	4 milliunits per minute

Amniotomy

The artificial rupture of membranes can be a favorable method of initiating uterine contractions and labor when the cervix is favorable. The fetal head should be well applied to the cervix and well engaged to reduce the risk of umbilical cord prolapse. The FHR should be monitored before and after the procedure; the color (clear or meconium stained) of the amniotic fluid should be documented, as well as the amount and odor of the fluid. Delivery achieved within 24 hours reduces the risk of chorioamnionitis. Therefore if spontaneous labor has not begun within 12 hours of rupture of membranes, the administration of oxytocin may be considered. The maternal temperature should be monitored per facility policy but no less frequently than every 4 hours after the rupture of membranes. Signs of infection should be documented and reported in an expeditious manner including fetal tachycardia, maternal fever, chills, or malodorous vaginal drainage.

Oxytocin Infusion: Augmentation or Induction of Labor

Oxytocin infusion may be used to either begin the labor process or to augment a labor that is progressing slowly because of inadequate uterine activity. Indications for induction include but are not limited to the following:

1. Pregnancy-induced hypertension
2. Premature rupture of membranes
3. Chorioamnionitis
4. Suspected fetal jeopardy as evidenced by biochemical or biophysical indications (e.g., fetal growth retardation, postterm gestation, and isoimmunization)
5. Maternal medical problems (e.g., diabetes mellitus, renal disease, and chronic obstructive pulmonary disease)

6. Fetal demise
7. Postterm gestation

Relative contraindications to induction include but are not limited to the following:

1. Placenta or vasa previa
2. Nonlongitudinal lie
3. Cord presentation
4. Presenting part above the pelvic inlet
5. Prior classical uterine incision
6. Active genital herpes infection
7. Pelvic structural deformities
8. Invasive cervical carcinoma

Assessment

Observations/Findings

Dysfunctional labor pattern (Table B-1)
Absence of cephalopelvic disproportion
Bishop Score (Table B-2)

Table B-1   Dysfunctional labor patterns

	Nullipara	Multipara
Prolonged latent phase	>21 hr	>14 hr
Protracted active phase	<1.2 cm/hr	<1.5 cm/hr
Secondary arrest: *no change*	>2 hr	>2 hr
Prolonged deceleration phase	>3 hr	>1 hr
Protracted descent	<1 cm/hr	<2 cm/hr
Arrest of descent	>1 hr	>$^1/_2$ hr

Table B-2   Bishop scoring system

	Score			
Area of Assessment	0	1	2	3
Station of presenting part	−3	−2	−1/0	+1/+2
Dilatation in cm	0	1-2	3-4	>5
Effacement in cm	>2.5	2	1	<0.5
Consistency	Firm	Medium	Soft	—
Position of os	Posterior	Central	Anterior	—

Laboratory/Diagnostic Studies

FHR-UA monitoring
Cephalopelvic disproportion (CPD) measurements
Ultrasound

Potential Complications

Fetal distress
   Late decelerations
   Prolonged deceleration
   Severe variable decelerations
Uterine hyperstimulation
   Contractions longer than 90 sec
   Contractions occurring more frequently than q2 min (tachysystole)
   Inadequate uterine relaxation: less than 30 sec between contractions
   Intrauterine resting tone: above 25 mm Hg pressure between contractions
   Sustained tetanic uterine contraction
Meconium passage
Maternal hypertension
Water intoxication
   Rising BP
   Edema of face and fingers and around the eyes
   Difficulty breathing
   Urinary output <30 to 50 ml/hr
Abruptio placentae: sudden, severe uterine pain
Rupture of vasa previa
Precipitate delivery
Hemorrhage
Shock
Uterine rupture
Amniotic fluid embolism

Medical Management

Baseline FHR-UC recording
Oxytocin infusion at a rate of 0.5 mU/min and increasing for desired results at 20- to 60-minute intervals in increments of 1 to 2 mU/min, not to exceed 20 mU/min
Continuous FHR-UA monitoring

Analgesia

Administer

Tocolytic agents for excessive uterine activity that persists after oxytocin is discontinued, supportive treatment provided (lateral position and oxygen by mask), and fetal distress is present.

Terbutaline 0.25 mg IV push or magnesium sulfate 4 grams, 10% solution over 15 to 20 minutes IV

Nursing Diagnoses/Interventions/Evaluation

■ NDX: Risk for injury related to augmentation of labor related to uterine hyperstimulation

See Care of Mother in First Stage of Labor (Appendix D)

Maintain complete bed rest

Ensure that physician is immediately available

Apply fetal monitoring; obtain baseline strip before starting IV oxytocin and before application of ripening agent

Place patient in comfortable position; lateral position is preferred

Always piggyback oxytocin solution into main IV line close to needle insertion site (10 U oxytocin in 1000 ml IV fluid = 10 mU/ml)

Administer oxytocin via a controlled infusion device as ordered

Monitor dose in mU/min q15 min and before each increase

Increase rate of oxytocic solution as ordered to produce contractions q2 to 3 min of 30 to 60 sec duration

Monitor patency of parenteral system

Check BP, P, and FHR q15 to 30 min or as ordered

Observe contractions for frequency, duration, strength, and relaxation q5 min for five times, then q15 to 30 min and prn

Administer analgesics as ordered

Assist in breathing and relaxation techniques

Measure intake and output q2h

Prepare for delivery as indicated

Reinforce physician's explanation of reason for augmentation or induction of labor

Expected outcome/evaluation

Mother and fetus are not compromised as a result of oxytocin infusion.

Patient Teaching

Reinforce physician's explanations

Discuss indications for procedure

Explain methodology of administration

Discuss expected effects of oxytocin induction/augmentation of labor

Explain differences between induction/augmentation and normal, spontaneous contractions

Ensure that patient and significant other verbalize understanding of procedure, indications for it, and expected effects.

Appendix C

Protocol for Management of Preterm Labor

Preterm Labor

Preterm labor is labor that occurs before completion of the thirty-seventh week of gestation. It is characterized by uterine contractions associated with changes in cervical parameters.

Contraindications to Tocolysis

Cervical dilatation > 4 cm
Ruptured membranes
Intrauterine infection
Severe intrauterine growth retardation
Clinically significant bleeding
Fetal anomalies incompatible with life

Assessment
Observations/findings

Uterine contractions
Every 10 min or less (6 to 8 uterine contractions/hour)
Lasting 30 sec or more
Progressive cervical dilatation: ≥50% effacement or ≥2 cm dilatation
Complaints of back pain or pressure
Possible spontaneous rupture of membranes

Therapy
Nifedipine therapy

Maternal effects
Slight flushing
Slight hypotension
Headache
Nausea
Peripheral edema
Periorbital edema
Syncope

Magnesium sulfate therapy

Maternal effects
  Flushing, sense of warmth
  Nasal stuffiness/congestion
  Headache
  Dizziness
  Respiratory depression
  Hypotension
  Hyporeflexia
  Nystagmus
  Nausea, vomiting
  Lethargy, fatigue
  Pulmonary edema
Fetal/neonatal effects
  Decreased muscle tone
  Respiratory depression
  Lethargy, drowsiness
  Lower Apgar scores with prolonged maternal treatment

Indomethacin therapy (Indocin)

Minimal gastrointestinal disturbance in mother
Fetal effects
  Possible premature closure of PDA (patent ductus areriosus)
  Possible impaired renal function resulting in oligohydramnios
Neonatal effect
  Temporary decrease in urine output less than 24 hours after
    last maternal dose

Terbutaline therapy

Maternal effects
  Tachycardia
  Palpitations
  Hypotension
  Arrhythmias
  Hypokalemia
  Chest pain
  Pulmonary edema
  Tremors
  Agitation
  Headache
  Elevated blood glucose
  Hyperlipidemia

Fetal/neonatal effects
  Fetal distress
  Tachycardia
  Bradycardia if severe maternal hypotension
  Neonatal hypotension
  Neonatal hypoglycemia
  Neonatal hypocalcemia
  Neonatal irritability

Ritodrine therapy

Maternal and fetal/neonatal effects (same as terbutaline)

Laboratory/Diagnostic Studies

Electronic fetal monitoring (EFM)
Fetoscope/Doppler
Urinalysis
CBC
Cervical cultures, including group B streptococcus
Amniocentesis to assess fetal lung maturity and presence of
  infection
Maternal and fetal baseline ECG
Electrolytes
Blood glucose
C-reactive protein (CRP)

Potential Complications

Compromised infant at birth
  Prematurity
  Small-for-gestational-age infant
  Respiratory distress syndrome

Medical Management

Bed rest may be indicated; semi-Fowler's position preferred
Continuous EFM and uterine contraction monitoring for a
  minimum of 1 hr
Home uterine monitoring as indicated by condition, uterine
  activity, fetal gestational age, and maternal compliance with
  this regimen
Laboratory tests as indicated
Monitor BP and TPR as indicated
IV fluids as indicated
Intake and output

Ultrasound for evaluation of placenta, fetal/uterine anomalies, and gestational age confirmation

Glucocorticoids as indicated

Tocolysis as indicated (nifedipine, magnesium sulfate, terbutaline, indomethacin, or ritodrine hydrochloride)

Antibiotics as indicated

Nursing Diagnoses/Interventions/ Evaluation

■ NDX: Risk for injury to fetus related to potential for preterm delivery; potential for injury to mother related to tocolysis therapy

Maintain complete bed rest in lateral position

Administer IV fluids as ordered

Note frequency, duration, and strength of contractions q15 min and prn; monitor uterine activity with tocotransducer (tocodynamometer) if available

Auscultate FHR q15 to 30 min or electronically monitor with ultrasound

Measure intake and output as ordered

Assist with amniocentesis and/or ultrasound if ordered

Administer any other medications, including corticosteroids, in exact dose, time, and route as ordered

Decrease frequency of nursing functions as patient's preterm labor is arrested

Continuous Labor

See Care of Mother in First Stage of Labor (Appendix D)

In addition

Prepare for high-risk infant

Notify neonatologist or pediatrician

Have resuscitative equipment ready for use

Plan to have infant's blood crossmatched if less than 32 weeks gestation

Monitor FHR electronically if possible

Assist physician with fetal blood sampling as indicated

Consider plotting labor dilation and descent on square-ruled graph paper (labor is usually rapid, but a high frequency of abnormal labors occur as well, such as Friedman curve)

Provide comfort measures before administering minimal doses of analgesics as ordered

Retain placenta for pathology as ordered

General Guidelines in the Use of Tocolytics

Limit tocolytic treatment to women with both cervical change and regular uterine contractions before 34-35 weeks gestation

If the first agent fails to produce tocolysis, use a second standard agent

Exercise caution with the combination of therapies

Use minimum amount of IV tocolytics for the shortest period of time

If tocolysis fails consider:

Placental abruption

Chorioamnionitis

Unsuspected uterine malformation

Use indomethacin and calcium blockers only in special circumstances

Respect maternal and fetal contraindications to tocolysis

Follow established protocols

Drug mixing

Amount of drug per ml

Administration precautions

Nifedipine

Oral administration

Administer 10 mg po, then 10 mg q6h or increase to 20 mg q6h to 8h

Sublingual administration

10 mg initially, then q20 min if needed to decrease uterine contractions (maximum dose is 40 mg/1 hour) followed by 10 mg po initiated 6 hours after the last sublingual capsule and then continue with the 10 mg oral regimen (may increase to 20 mg q6h if uterine contractions increase)

Magnesium sulfate

Maintain patent IV access

Administer 3 to 6 g IV in a 10% solution over 15 to 30 min for initial dose as ordered

Continue and monitor IV infusion titrated according to uterine response and side effects (i.e., 2 g/hr)

Watch for symptoms of toxicity; discontinue, administer oxygen
therapy, and notify physician if toxicity occurs
Respiratory depression
Hypotension
Absence of deep tendon reflexes
Keep antidote for magnesium sulfate toxicity (10% calcium
gluconate) at bedside
Monitor and decrease dosage after 24 hr or when uterine con-
tractions subside as ordered
Check vital signs and DTRs q30 min to 1 hr
Continue to monitor uterine activity
Monitor intake and output q1h; should be at least 30 ml urine
per hour
Auscultate lungs q4h to 8h for presence of fluid
Monitor fetus with EFM as ordered
Check fetal heart rate with vital signs if no EFM is done
Monitor magnesium sulfate levels
Obtain baseline electrolytes and calcium levels by venipuncture

Indomethacin

Oral administration for SHORT TERM USE ONLY (48 hours)
Initial dose 50 mg po followed by 25 mg po q4 hours for 24-
48 hours
Note: Physician may order sucralfate (Carafate) 1 g 30 min
before all doses of indomethacin

β_2 Adrenergic Agents (Terbutaline and Ritodrine)
Terbutaline

Parenteral administration
Administer loading dose of 0.25 mg slowly
For continued therapy add 15 mg terbutaline to 250 ml of 5
DW or NS (this will deliver 60 μg/ml)
Give 5 μg/min and increase dose in 5 μg increments q10
minutes until tocolysis is achieved or until 55 μg/min is
reached
Oral therapy
Administer first dose before discontinuing parenteral therapy
Dosage 2.5 to 5.0 mg q4h po until 36 weeks gestation
Subcutaneous administration

Administer 0.25 mg SQ, and repeat same dose in 30 min if
uterine contractions persist

For continued therapy give 0.25 mg SQ every 4 hours for 24
hours and then switch to oral therapy or per physician order

If birth occurs quickly after the administration of terbutaline,
monitor closely and be prepared to manage uterine atony
and postpartum hemorrhage

Ritodrine hydrochloride

Obtain laboratory data as ordered (may include CBC, electrolytes, and glucose)

Place in lateral position during infusion

Monitor maternal electrocardiogram (ECG) as ordered

Administer ritodrine (usually 50 µg/min) via infusion pump or
controller with drug piggybacked into main IV line, being
careful not to exceed maximum dosage of 350 µg/min

Monitor rate and dosage and increase by 50 µg/min q10 min
based on maternal and fetal responses as ordered

Guidelines for terbutaline and ritodrine therapy

Do not increase dose and/or discontinue terbutaline or ritodrine if patient demonstrates unacceptable side effects: if
maternal heart rate exceeds 140 beats/min, if fetal tachycardia of 180 beats/min or greater persists, if systolic blood
pressure is < 90 mm Hg or more than a 20% decrease, if diastolic BP is < 40 mm Hg

Check BP, P, and FHR q10 min while increasing dosage, then
q30 min while patient is receiving IV maintenance dose

Monitor FHR and uterine contractions continuously if possible

Report undesirable side effects, including headache and palpitations, to physician

Continue to maintain IV infusion for 12 hr after arrest of labor,
using smallest dose possible to maintain tocolysis

Adjust dosage of tocolytic agent for patients with diurnal patterns of uterine activity

Auscultate lungs q8h to check for fluid overload

Monitor intake and output q1h

Initiate oral therapy 30 min before discontinuing IV therapy
as ordered

Decrease frequency of nursing functions as preterm labor is arrested

Expected outcome/evaluation

Preterm delivery is avoided; there are no maternal complications of tocolysis therapy

■ NDX: Risk for situational low self-esteem related to perceptions and expectations of pregnancy and delivery

Encourage patient to verbalize fears and concerns
Note and document
    Minimal eye contact
    Self-defeating statements and/or behaviors
    Overt expressions of guilt or blame
    Negativity or inadequacy in actions or verbal communications
    Demonstrations of anger
Include significant other in discussions
Provide factual information about placement of blame for initiation and continuation of uterine contractions
Provide positive feedback and encouragement to patient for seeking early interventions

Expected outcome/evaluation

Patient verbalizes positive feelings about self

■ NDX: Pain related to uterine contractions

Use nonpharmacological measures when appropriate
    Positioning
    Muscular relaxation techniques
    Breathing techniques
    Distraction techniques
Eliminate or minimize other factors that could contribute to pain
    Encourage frequent voiding
    Explain all procedures before executing them
    Answer all questions if possible
    Offer choices to allow for control as patient is able
    Keep patient and significant other informed of changes in labor and fetal status
Explain reasons why analgesic agents may not be appropriate
    Effect on fetal heart rate
    Possible masking of contractions
    Combined side effects of tocolytic agents and analgesia

Provide positive reinforcement and touch as appropriate

Plan nursing care to provide rest periods to promote comfort, sleep, and relaxation

Assess and document stress-contributing factors to perception of pain

Assess and document q30 min

Frequency and length of contractions

Location of pain

Intensity and duration of pain

Expected outcome/evaluation

Patient will verbalize decreasing or more tolerable discomfort

Patient Teaching/Discharge Planning

Explain arrested labor

Emphasize importance of maintaining rest

Emphasize importance of avoiding intercourse, douching, or nipple stimulation, including preparation of breasts for breast-feeding

Teach name of medication, dosage, frequency of administration, purpose, and toxic side effects

Teach or reinforce instructions if patient will be monitored at home with periodic modem transmission of uterine activity

Emphasize importance of having supportive person to perform housekeeping, cooking, and child care tasks

Discuss signs of labor to report to physician

Emphasize importance of follow-up medical care

Discuss development and gestational stage of fetus

Appendix D

Guidelines for Care of the Patient in Labor: First Stage and Second Stage

First Stage of Labor

Early labor dilatation of 0 to 4 cm with mild to moderate irregular contractions

Active labor dilatation of 4 cm with moderate to strong regular contractions q2 min to 5 min

Transitional labor dilatation of 8 cm to complete dilatation with strong contractions

Assessment

Observations/findings

Rupture of membranes
· Early labor
  Surge of energy and activity
  Talking frequently
  Mildly anxious
  Fear of isolation
  Uterine contractions 5 to 30 minutes apart lasting 10 to 40 seconds
  Effaced 0-50%
  Station 0 to −2
Active labor
  More focused on the progress of labor
  Less talkative
  Increased dependency on significant other or caregiver
  More apprehensive
  Uterine contractions 2 to 4 minutes apart lasting 30 to 50 seconds
  Effaced 50-80%
  Station 0 to +1

Transitional labor
    Increased bloody show
    Uterine contractions 2 to 3 minutes apart lasting 50 to 60 seconds
    Effaced 100%
    Station +1 to +2
    Nausea and vomiting
    Irritability
    Loss of coping mechanism
    Hiccups and/or belching
    Trembling and/or shaking of legs
    Chilling
    Perspiration
    Rectal pressure
    Urge to push
    Hypersensitive abdomen

Laboratory/diagnostic studies

Baseline laboratory tests
CBC with differential
Blood type, Rh, Indirect Coombs
VDRL serology
Chemistries
Rubella Titer
Hepatitis screen
Varicella Titer
Urinalysis
Cultures as indicated by history of signs and symptoms
Ultrasound/x-ray examination as indicated
Acid-base monitoring

Potential complications

Nonreassuring findings
    Fetal tachycardia: above 160 bpm
    Fetal bradycardia: below 120 bpm
    Meconium-stained amniotic fluid
    Foul-smelling amniotic fluid
Fetal hyperactivity
Monitored labor
    Severe variable decelerations: <70 bpm for more than 30 sec
    Uncorrectable, repetitive late decelerations of any magnitude

Absence of variability
Prolonged deceleration
Unstable FHR; sinusoidal pattern
Supine hypotension syndrome
Inadequate uterine relaxation
Contractions lasting longer than 90 sec
Relaxation between contractions less than 30 sec
Arrest of labor
Amnionitis secondary to prolonged rupture of membranes
Elevated temperature
Distended bladder
Dehydration
Hemorrhage
Prolapsed umbilical cord
Abruptio placentae

Medical Management

Laboratory tests as indicated
IV fluids as indicated
Prenatal chart and previous medical chart ordered to labor and
delivery unit
Vital sign monitoring according to facility policy
Analgesia as indicated
Preparation for selected/indicated anesthesia by anesthesiolo-
gist/nurse anesthetist
Fetal heart rate-uterine contraction (FHR-UC) monitoring

Maternal-Fetal Assessment Frequencies

Low risk patients
Temperature and pulse q4h (if ROM then q1 hour)
Blood pressure q1h
Evaluate and record the FHR and UA every 30 min in the
active phase of the first stage of labor and every 15 min
during the second stage
High risk patients
Temperature, pulse, and blood pressure q1h or more frequently
if situation necessitates
Evaluate and record the FHR and UA every 15 min in the active
phase of the first stage of labor and every 5 min during the
second stage

Nursing Diagnoses/Interventions/ Evaluation

■ NDX: Risk for injury to mother related to physiological processes of labor and to infection secondary to contamination

Review prenatal history for any risk factors

Check temperature q2h after rupture of membranes

Consider plotting cervical dilation and fetal descent over time on square-ruled graph paper (Friedman curve)

Give enema in early labor if ordered

Administer clear liquids as ordered

Monitor intake and output

Have patient void q2h and prn

Check urine for glucose and protein

Maintain complete bed rest in position of comfort if membranes are ruptured, especially if presenting part is not yet engaged; otherwise, patient may ambulate as tolerated

Allow patient up to bathroom as ordered if presenting part is well applied to cervix

Initiate lactated Ringer's solution or other IV solution as ordered

Prehydrate with 500 to 1000 ml of fluid before anesthetic procedure as ordered

Maintain dosing of prelabor medications or drugs as ordered (i.e., anticonvulsants, antihypertensives, or methadone)

Expected outcome/evaluation

Patient does not experience any injury related to labor as evidenced by adequate hydration, skin turgor, voiding pattern (absence of distended bladder)

There is no fever or other evidence of infection

■ NDX: Pain and anxiety related to intensity of uterine contractions and fear of the unknown

Active labor

Offer back rub qh and prn between contractions

Apply pressure to sacrum as needed prn during contractions

Explain all procedures

Provide anticipatory guidance to the normal process of labor

Apply cool compress to forehead prn

Maintain dry pads under buttocks; remove moist or wet pads immediately

Assist with breathing techniques and teach significant other to assist patient

Praise patient and significant other on their performance of relaxation techniques

Change gown and linen as necessary

Turn off bright overhead lights when not needed

Clip call bell to bottom sheet within easy reach to ensure that staff is promptly notified of patient's needs

Relieve discomfort with medication as ordered

Assist physician with local or regional anesthetic; take BP and P q10 min for three times after anesthetic and until stabilized

Avoid talking to patient during contractions

Reposition patient q30 min and prn; lateral position is preferred

Transitional phase of labor

Encourage deep ventilation before and after each contraction when patient is in active labor and during transition period

Have patient avoid urge to push by panting and/or blowing in rapid sequence with contractions until completely dilated

Have emesis basin readily available

Have patient void to ensure empty bladder

Cover feet with blanket or have patient wear socks if chilling occurs

Tell patient that the transition stage usually lasts no more than 1 to 2 hr and then she will be allowed to push and deliver infant

Palpate abdomen very lightly and only as often as necessary if abdomen is hypersensitive

Avoid having persons in labor room who are not directly caring for patient

Accept aggression or other coping behaviors; avoid negative comments

Avoid unnecessary talking or expression of feelings to meet own needs

Focus on patient and support her

    Calm voice

    Touch

    Positive reinforcement after contractions

Expected outcome/evaluation

Patient experiences manageable pain and minimal anxiety as evidenced by verbalization of same

Complies with assistive directions by staff

Has continuing positive interaction with significant other/ family

■ NDX: Altered oral mucous membrane related to mouth breathing

Administer oral hygiene qh and prn between contractions

Suck on ice chips, wet washcloths, or sour lollipops unless contraindicated

Rinse mouth with water and/or mouthwash

Apply petroleum jelly or antichapping lipsticks to dry lips prn

Expected outcome/evaluation

Patient does not experience disruption in tissue layers of oral cavity

■ NDX: Risk for injury to fetus related to uterine contractions of labor and/or uteroplacental insufficiency

Note frequency, duration, and strength of contractions q30 min to 60 min and prn in early labor; increase to q15 min to 30 min in active labor

Auscultate FHR immediately after uterine contractions, preferably for one full minute if not electronically monitored in first stage of labor (q15 min to 30 min and prn)

Check BP qh and prn

Note presence of variability if electronically monitored

Assess for decrease of variability expected from administration of narcotics and fetal sleep cycle

Check T, P, and R q2h to 4h and prn

Auscultate FHR immediately after membranes rupture or amniotomy is done

Turn mother to lateral position, increase rate of plain IV, administer 100% oxygen by face mask, and notify physician immediately if nonreassuring pattern is evident by auscultation or electronic fetal monitoring.

Expected outcome/evaluation

Patient delivers an infant in good condition at birth with Apgar score ≥8 at 5 min of age

■ NDX: Anxiety related to lack of knowledge and uncertainty about what to expect during labor

Allay anxiety as much as possible by doing the following:
  Explain reasons for performing all procedures
  Accommodate birth plans of patient and family as appropriate
  Encourage spouse or significant other to remain with the patient to provide support during labor
  Let spouse or significant other listen to fetal heart tones with stethoscope, fetoscope, or ultrasound stethoscope
  Provide supportive care based on patient's knowledge of the labor process
  Inform waiting family members and friends of patient's progress, and let the patient know that they are interested in her
  Reduce environmental stimuli that may contribute to anxiety and tension; provide a relaxed, restful atmosphere
  At appropriate intervals reassure the patient that labor is progressing and that both patient and infant are doing fine

Expected outcome/evaluation

Patient verbalizes understanding of process of labor and rationale for procedures
Is supported by significant other in coping with anxiety

Procedural Care of the Patient During the Second Stage of Labor

The stage of expulsion of the fetus, placenta, and membranes from the mother at birth after complete dilatation of the cervix

Assessment

Observations/findings

  Involuntary bearing down
  Pushing
  Grunting sounds
  Extreme anxiety
  Vomiting episode
  Involuntary shaking of legs
  Perspiration between nose and upper lip
  Increase in bloody show
  Patient stating, "Baby is coming"
  Desire to defecate, fear of "making a mess"

Prolonged second stage
    More than 1 hr for multigravidas
    More than 2 hr for primigravidas

Laboratory/diagnostic studies

Electronic fetal monitoring
Cord blood: gases, pH, and other tests as ordered

Potential complications/risks

High-risk delivery
Abruptio placentae
Difficult delivery
    Shoulder dystocia
    Breech presentation
    Cephalopelvic disproportion
Forceps delivery
Vacuum extraction
Cesarean section
Infant bruising, fractures

Nursing Procedures
Care during delivery

Provide for 1:1 staffing ratio
Auscultate FHR q5 min and/or after each push if electronic
    monitor is not used (if electronic monitor was used continu-
    ously during labor, then it should be continued in the delivery
    room until the time of delivery)
Check BP and P q10 min and prn
Pad stirrups
Administer oxygen by snug face mask at 10 to 12 L/min as ordered
Understand that an upright position with lateral tilt is preferred
    while pushing
Assist with breathing techniques
    Ventilation before and after each contraction
    Breathing technique and open glottis gentle pushing with con-
        tractions
Observe perineum while pushing
Notify physician if second stage is prolonged
Prepare perineum according to hospital procedure
Place nurse, spouse, and/or labor coach at head of delivery table
    to encourage patient during delivery process
Encourage long, sustained pushing rather than frequent short pushes

Encourage complete relaxation between contractions

Reassure patient that she is doing well and is advancing the infant with each push

Apply cool, moist cloth to forehead as needed

Have DeLee suction catheter available and ready to use if meconium-stained amniotic fluid is present

Plan for suctioning of naso-oropharynx after delivery of fetal head and before delivery of thorax to prevent meconium aspiration

Assist physician or nurse-midwife as needed

Immediate postdelivery care

Permit mother to inspect infant as soon as possible

Place infant on maternal abdomen to provide skin-to-skin contact if delivery room is warm

Defer neonatal eye therapy for 1 to 2 hr after birth to promote eye contact with mother

Check BP and P q10 min to 15 min for four times and prn

Add oxytocic drug as ordered to parenteral fluids

Palpate fundus, noting location and tonus q5 min to 10 min for four times

Administer perineal care before removing legs from stirrups

Place sterile perineal pad and/or pad under buttocks before transporting patient to recovery area

Place ice pack on episiotomy unless otherwise ordered

Maintain mother's warmth with blankets as needed

Place radiant heat warmer over upper part of mother's bed or place dry, warmly blanketed infant next to mother so that she can visually inspect, touch, and/or breastfeed nude infant while preventing neonatal heat loss

Let mother and spouse and/or labor coach be with infant in delivery area, providing them with as much privacy as feasible unless this is contraindicated by maternal or fetal condition

Encourage mother to freely express her feelings about herself and her infant

Explain that behaviors manifested in labor are normal and there is no reason to apologize if mother is apologetic for behavior while in labor

Appendix E

Selected Pattern Interpretation

Fetal Tachycardia

SIGNAL SOURCE   Spiral electrode and tocotransducer

FHR   Baseline: 190 to 200 bpm

Variability: Average

Periodic changes: No significant changes; a mild variable deceleration occurs in panel 30266.

UTERINE ACTIVITY   Frequency: 2 to 2½ minutes

Duration: 30 to 40 seconds

Note the wide excursion vertical lines, probably caused by electrical "noise" or interference. If these lines were more frequent and consistent, they would suggest a fetal dysrhythmia.

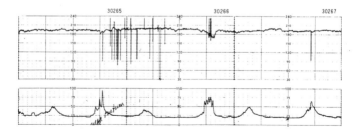

Fetal Bradycardia

SIGNAL SOURCE   Spiral electrode and intrauterine catheter

FHR   Baseline: 110 bpm

                       Variability: Average

                       Periodic changes: No significant
                         changes

UTERINE ACTIVITY   Frequency: 3 to 3½ minutes

                       Duration: 50 to 60 seconds

                       Intensity: 50 to 65 mm Hg

                       Resting tone: 5 mm Hg

Flat Baseline

SIGNAL SOURCE	Spiral electrode and tocotransducer
FHR	Baseline: 140 to 150 bpm
	Variability: Minimal
	Periodic changes: No significant changes

This fetus was 3 weeks overdue and later delivered spontaneously with a meconium-stained placenta, birth weight of 4067 g (9 lb 1¼ oz), and Apgar scores of 4 at 1 minute and 7 at 5 minutes of age.

UTERINE ACTIVITY	Contractions are either not present, or the tocotransducer is misplaced. The uterine activity demonstrated here is normal for the patient who is not in labor. Respiratory movements are clearly seen.

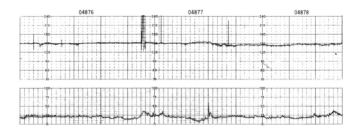

Acceleration of FHR with UC

SIGNAL SOURCE   Spiral electrode and tocotransducer

FHR   Baseline: 140 to 150 bpm

                        Variability: Average

                        Periodic changes: Acceleration of FHR
                            occurs with each contraction. The
                            amplitude of the acceleration is
                            markedly increased when the patient
                            pushes with contractions.

UTERINE ACTIVITY   Frequency: 2½ minutes

                        Duration: 40 to 50 seconds

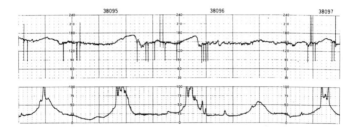

Acceleration of FHR with UC

SIGNAL SOURCE	Spiral electrode and intrauterine catheter
FHR	Baseline: 130 bpm
	Variability: Average
	Periodic changes: Acceleration of fetal heart rate occurs with each contraction and with fetal movement as evidenced by the spikes in the UA panel just before the two middle contractions. Sometimes acceleration of FHR with contractions or before contractions makes the FHR look as if late decelerations are occurring, when given a casual glance. Therefore it is important to identify the baseline rate and note the timing of the acceleration or deceleration in relation to the uterine contraction.
UTERINE ACTIVITY	Frequency: 3 to 3½ minutes
	Duration: 60 to 70 seconds
	Intensity: Probably 75 to 85 mm Hg
	Resting tone: Probably 30 to 35 mm Hg

The strain gauge has not been opened to room air and calibrated. The resting tone and intensity of the contractions are most likely much lower than are reflected in this tracing.

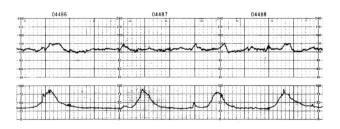

Early Decelerations

SIGNAL SOURCE	Ultrasound and tocotransducer
FHR	Baseline: 120 bpm
	Variability: Not specific with ultrasound but probably minimal
	Periodic changes: Consistent early decelerations occur with each contraction because of head compression.
UTERINE ACTIVITY	Frequency: 2 to 3 minutes
	Duration: 40 to 50 seconds

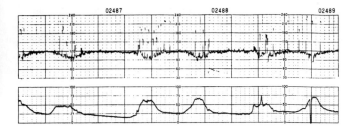

Mild Variable Decelerations

SIGNAL SOURCE   Spiral electrode and tocotransducer

FHR   Baseline: 140 bpm

Variability: Average

Periodic changes: Mild variable decelerations in FHR occur with each
contraction. This frequently occurs
with pushing and signals the second
stage of labor.

UTERINE ACTIVITY   Frequency: 1½ to 2 minutes

Duration: 30 to 40 seconds

Spikes of uterine pressure above 50 mm Hg indicate maternal
pushing.

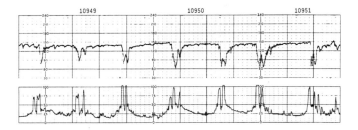

Fetal Cardiac Dysrhythmia

SIGNAL SOURCE	Spiral electrode and intrauterine catheter
FHR	Baseline: 170 bpm; the vertical excursions from the baseline indicate a cardiac arrhythmia. If they were less frequent and more random, they would suggest electrical interference or "noise." Clinically, this pattern is not a cause for consideration of termination of labor. Most fetal cardiac dysrhythmias disappear after birth and are not considered a sign of fetal distress.
	Variability: Minimal
UTERINE ACTIVITY	Frequency: 1½ to 6 minutes
	Duration: 50 to 60 seconds
	Intensity: 50+ mm Hg with patient pushing
	Resting tone: 10 mm Hg

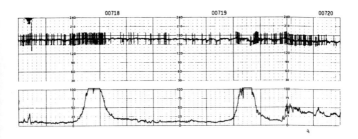

External Mode of Monitoring— Clear Tracing

SIGNAL SOURCE   Ultrasound and tocotransducer

FHR   Baseline: 140 bpm

Variability: Not specific with ultrasound but probably average

Periodic changes: No significant changes

UTERINE ACTIVITY   Frequency: 2 to 2½ minutes

Duration: 30 to 50 seconds

Note the zigzag respiratory movements of the uterine activity panel.

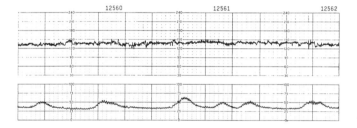

Loose Spiral Electrode with Complete Cervical Dilatation

SIGNAL SOURCE   Spiral electrode and tocotransducer

FHR   Baseline: 136 bpm in panel 55986. The
                         sudden loss of FHR signal in panel
                         55987 is due to loose spiral electrode
                         (lead) since complete dilatation has
                         occurred. The actual FHR was then
                         auscultated at 136 bpm, which is
                         consistent with the previously known
                         baseline.

                         Variability: Unable to determine

                         Periodic changes: Unable to determine

UTERINE ACTIVITY   Frequency: 2½ to 3 minutes

                         Duration: 50 to 90 seconds

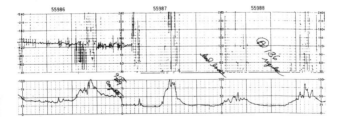

Coupling of Uterine Contractions

SIGNAL SOURCE	Spiral electrode and intrauterine catheter
FHR	Baseline: 130 bpm
	Variability: Average
	Periodic changes: No significant changes
UTERINE ACTIVITY	Frequency: 1½ to 4½ minutes
	Duration: 40 seconds
	Intensity: 60 mm Hg
	Resting tone: 5 mm Hg

Laboring patterns vary among individuals. Note the characteristic coupling of uterine contractions in this tracing.

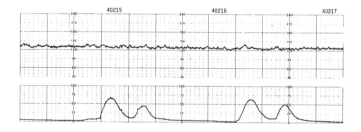

Appendix F

Position Statement of the Association of Women's Health, Obstetric, and Neonatal Nurses (AWHONN)

ISSUE: NURSING RESPONSIBILITIES IN IMPLEMENTING INTRAPARTUM FETAL HEART RATE MONITORING

The primary goal of perinatal care is to ensure optimal maternal and neonatal outcomes. The intrapartum period represents a time of risk for the mother and the fetus. Assessment of fetal heart rate (FHR) has been recognized as a vital aspect in the evaluation of fetal well-being in response to the stresses of labor and birth.

Auscultation and electronic fetal monitoring (EFM) are the basic techniques used to assess FHR. Each method has its advantages and limitations, necessitating individualized decision making for appropriate use. The method of FHR monitoring selected and the frequency of FHR evaluation should be based on consideration of maternal-fetal risk factors and the availability of nursing personnel who are skilled in the monitoring techniques. The patient's preference regarding the method of FHR monitoring should be taken into consideration.

Nurses who perform FHR monitoring are responsible for their actions and will be held to the established standards of care as defined by their professional organizations, the standards of practice in their institutions, and the scope of practice as defined by their nurse practice act.

Methodology

Auscultation. Auscultation of the FHR is an auditory assessment procedure that, when properly performed, allows evaluation of FHR both during and immediately following the stress of a uterine contraction. Auscultation between contractions establishes the baseline

Approved by Executive Board, October 1988. Revised February 1992.

FHR. Auscultation as a primary technique of FHR surveillance requires a thorough knowledge of the basic principles of the fetal heart and uterine physiology and pathophysiology. Clinical experience in the recognition of and the response to significant FHR changes is required. Validation of competency in the use of this technique must be in accordance with established institutional policy.

Intermittent auscultation of the fetal heart with a 1:1 nurse-patient ratio at 15-minute intervals during the active phase of the first stage of labor and at 5-minute intervals during the second stage has been shown to be equivalent to EFM (American Academy of Pediatrics and the American College of Obstetricians and Gynecologists [ACOG], 1992). For low-risk patients, the suggested auscultation frequency is 30-minute intervals in active first-stage labor and 15-minute intervals in second-stage labor (NAACOG, 1990). For high-risk patients, the suggested auscultation frequency is 15-minute intervals in active first-stage labor and 5-minute intervals in second-stage labor (NAACOG, 1990). Therefore, if auscultation is prescribed as the primary technique of FHR surveillance in the second stage of labor, a minimum of a 1:1 nurse-fetus ratio is required.

Electronic Fetal Monitoring. EFM is an auditory and visual assessment procedure that provides data for the evaluation of uterine activity and fetal heart responses, including baseline heart rate, variability, and fetal heart rate change over time. Further, EFM produces a printed record. The use of EFM requires knowledge of its equipment and thorough knowledge of the basic principles of the fetal heart and uterine physiology and pathophysiology. Nurses who use EFM must be able to recognize FHR patterns, variability, and uterine activity.

Fetal monitoring patterns have been given descriptive names, for example, accelerations and early, late, and variable decelerations. Nurses should use these terms in written chart documentation and verbal communication. Deviations from a normal heart rate pattern should be documented. When such changes in a FHR pattern occur, the nurse also should document a subsequent return to a normal pattern.

The patient's medical record should include observations and assessments of fetal heart rate and characteristics of uterine activity, as well as specific actions taken when changes in fetal heart rate patterns are observed. The monitor tracing is a legal part of the medical record and should include identifying information about the patient, as well as times and events related to the patient's ongoing care.

After identification of a nonreassuring pattern, the nurse is responsible for initiating and documenting appropriate nursing interventions as indicated by the pattern identified and for notifying a physician or certified nurse-midwife. Documentation of such notification should be entered in the patient's medical record. The nurse can expect the physician or certified nurse-midwife to respond after being notified of a nonreassuring pattern. An institutional policy should be established for the nurse to follow in the event that the physician or certified nurse-midwife is unable to respond in a timely fashion.

Core competencies in FHR monitoring have been published by NAACOG (1991). Competency validation of this expertise must be in accordance with established institutional policy (NAACOG, 1988).

Evaluation and Documentation

The institution should establish policies, procedures, and protocols that define evaluation and documentation of FHR monitoring. In developing policies, procedures, and protocols, the institution should address the following:

- method(s) for assessment (EFM, auscultation, or a combination of both)
- maternal-fetal risk factors
- stage of labor
- frequency of assessment
- qualifications of health-care providers performing assessments
- nurse-fetus ratios

Documentation of the evaluation of FHR monitoring information during labor is applicable regardless of the method of monitoring selected and may be accomplished in narrative nurses' notes and/or by the use of comprehensive flow sheets at the time of assessment. Documentation also may be achieved by the use of abbreviated nurses' notes with follow-up summary nurses' notes at intervals specified by institutional policy. The format for abbreviated notes may include initiating the EFM tracing, annotating the EFM tracing, or annotating basic flow sheets.

Suggested frequencies for interval evaluation of FHR information using auscultation have been addressed. For high-risk patients being monitored with auscultation during the active phase of the first stage and during the second stage of labor, intervals for both the evaluation and recording of FHR information are suggested at 15 and 5 minutes, respectively (NAACOG, 1990). For the same group of patients being monitored electronically, evaluation of the tracing is suggested at the same intervals (ACOG, 1989). For low-risk patients being monitored with auscultation, the suggested intervals for evaluation and recording are at 30 and 15 minutes in the active phase of the first and the second stage of labor, respectively. The standard practice for low-risk patients being monitored electronically is to evaluate and record the FHR at least every 30 minutes following a contraction in the active phase of the first stage of labor and at least every 15 minutes in the second stage of labor (ACOG, 1989).

Evaluation of FHR information may take place at the intervals suggested above or more frequently as necessitated by the individual patient-care situation. Written documentation of these FHR evaluations, however, may occur at longer intervals in narrative, abbreviated, and/or summary formats, in accordance with institutional policy and procedure.

Conflict Resolution

The potential for conflict exists in terms of professional judgment and decision making regarding which method of monitoring is best for a particular patient in a given situation. Institutional policies, procedures, and protocols must provide a mechanism that will allow nurses the flexibility to decline to implement the prescribed method of FHR monitoring if any question exists regarding the ability to meet the required staffing ratios or if the methodology is beyond the individual nurse's expertise. Ultimately, the responsibility for implementing the prescribed method of FHR monitoring remains with the prescriber. In the event of differences of opinion among professionals regarding the ability to implement the prescribed method, the established institutional policy for resolution of conflict should be followed.

References

American Academy of Pediatrics and American College of Obstetricians and Gynecologists: *Guidelines for perinatal care,* ed 3, Washington, DC, 1992, The Academy and The College.

Nurses Association of the American College of Obstetricians and Gynecologists: *OGN nursing practice resource: Fetal heart auscultation,* Washington, DC, 1990, The Association.

Nurses Association of the American College of Obstetricians and Gynecologists: *Nursing practice competencies and educational guidelines: Antepartum fetal surveillance and intrapartum fetal heart monitoring,* Washington, DC, 1991, The Association.

Nurses Association of the American College of Obstetricians and Gynecologists: *Essentials of electronic fetal monitoring competency validation,* Washington, DC, 1991, The Association.

American College of Obstetricians and Gynecologists: *ACOG technical bulletin: Intrapartum fetal heart rate monitoring,* Number 132, Washington, DC, 1989, The College and The Association.

Appendix G

Nursing Practice Competencies and Educational Guidelines: Antepartum Fetal Surveillance and Intrapartum Fetal Heart Monitoring

This document outlines specific areas of competency expected of each nurse whose practice includes the use of fetal surveillance techniques in assessing, promoting, and evaluating maternal and fetal well-being during the antepartum and intrapartum periods. This document also provides guidelines for educational programs to prepare nurses for practice, using fetal heart monitoring techniques. Educational programs include both core and ongoing instruction. A core instructional program includes the essential theoretical and clinical principles to achieve minimal competency. Ongoing instruction includes additional theoretical and clinical education to maintain competency. Nurses are encouraged to refer to institutional policy and related nurse practice acts to determine the scope of nursing practice regarding fetal heart monitoring and antepartum fetal surveillance in individual practice settings.

Antepartum Fetal Surveillance
Nursing Practice Competencies

Nurses with responsibility for performing antepartum fetal surveillance should demonstrate competency in the application and use of external electronic and auscultatory fetal monitoring equipment and the interpretation of data. Before assuming responsibility for antepartum monitoring, the nurse should be able to do the following:
1. Describe antepartum testing criteria and indications for testing, for example, high-risk pregnancy

From NAACOG: The Organization for Obstetric, Gynecologic and Neonatal Nurses, 409 12th Street SW, Washington, DC 20024-21; ©1986 by the Nurses' Association of the American College of Obstetricians and Gynecologists. All rights reserved; and ©1991 by NAACOG: The Organization for Obstetric, Gynecologic and Neonatal Nurses.

2. Provide patient education regarding the procedure and its purpose
3. Prepare the patient; perform complete assessment, including Leopold's maneuvers; palpate the fundus; apply the external electronical fetal monitor
4. Recognize contraindications to the use of oxytocin and nipple stimulation
5. Conduct the prescribed antepartum test
6. Implement interventions per protocol for nonreassuring findings
7. Communicate the content of electronic fetal monitoring data for final interpretation in accordance with institutional policy
8. Document appropriate entries in the written or computerized patient record and the electronic fetal monitoring tracing or storage disk
9. Discontinue electronic fetal monitoring according to institutional policy, procedure, and protocol
10. Communicate appropriate follow-up information to the patient

Biophysical profile components, including fetal movement, tone, breathing, and amniotic fluid volume, and other ultrasound assessments, such as fetal position and placental grading and location, may be performed in accordance with institutional policy and the nurse practice act after appropriate educational and clinical instruction in the technique.

Educational Guidelines

Three to four hours of didactic instruction specific to antepartum fetal heart monitoring is considered the minimum requirement. Didactic instruction should be followed by supervised clinical experience before independent nursing practice. The period of supervised clinical experience required to achieve competency varies with the individual and the practice setting.

Additional didactic instruction and supervised clinical experience specific to antepartum fetal surveillance with ultrasound will vary with the individual and the practice setting.

Didactic content outline

I. Elements of antepartum fetal surveillance
   A. Maternal-fetal physiology
   B. Indication for testing
   C. Methods and interpretation
      1. Nonstress test

   2. Contraction stress test
      (a) Spontaneous
      (b) Nipple stimulation
      (c) Oxytocin
   D. Contraindications for use of oxytocin and nipple stimulation
      1. Ultrasound evaluation, biophysical profile, and other similar noninvasive assessments, according to institutional policy and nurse practice acts
 II. Patient education
   A. Indication for testing
   B. Test procedure
   C. Test results
   D. Follow-up
III. Nursing accountability
   A. Policies, procedures, and protocols
   B. Standards of practice
   C. Follow-up: interpretation and reporting protocol
   D. Documentation in the written or computerized patient record and on the electronic fetal monitor tracing or storage disk
   E. Legal and ethical issues
   F. Lines of authority and responsibility (chain of command)

Clinical learning experiences and evaluation

The sequence and specific nature of clinical learning experiences can be adapted to accommodate clinical instructors' or preceptors' styles and individual learners' needs.
A. Practice sessions should include a policy, procedure, and protocol manual review and also may include the following:
   1. Electronic fetal monitor tracing review sessions
   2. Small group discussion/case studies
   3. Clinical conferences (multidisciplinary)
   4. Role-play situations
   5. Videotaped observation and follow-up discussion
   6. Computer simulation
   7. One-to-one tutorial
   8. Self-study
B. Practicum
   1. Demonstration with return demonstration of equipment, setup, application, and calibration

2. Demonstration with return demonstration of equipment maintenance
C. Clinical application of the nursing process under the supervision of the instructor or preceptor
   1. Instruction of the patient and family
   2. Selection of method of assessment
   3. Application of technology (including calibration)
   4. Recognition of technology errors and limitations
   5. Formulation of a nursing diagnosis or nursing problem
   6. Intervention
   7. Documentation in the written or computerized patient record and on the electronic fetal monitor tracing or storage disk
   8. Evaluation and follow-up

Competency Validation

Evaluation of didactic and clinical learning validates competency. Evaluation can be ongoing during the learning process or conducted at the conclusion of the learning experiences. The components that comprise validation include the following:
A. Written or verbal exercises such as
   1. Examination
   2. Case study analysis
   3. Electronic fetal monitor tracing interpretation sessions
   4. Interpretation of hospital policies, procedures, and protocols
   5. Identification of appropriate lines of authority and responsibility (chain of command)
B. Observation by instructor or preceptor of nurse providing patient care in fetal heart monitoring clinical situations
C. Documentation of competency in the fetal surveillance technique before the nurse functions independently

Intrapartum Fetal Heart Monitoring
Nursing Practice Competencies

To function competently in the use of intrapartum fetal heart monitoring, the nurse should demonstrate competency in the application and use of auscultatory and electronic fetal monitoring equipment and interpretation of data. The intrapartum nurse should therefore be able to do the following:

A. Implement the appropriate fetal heart monitoring method based on patient status, hospital policy, and current standards of practice recommended by professional organizations

B. Explain the principles of the chosen method of fetal heart monitoring to the patient and her support person(s)

C. Identify the limitations of information produced by each method of monitoring

D. Demonstrate competency in fetal heart monitoring by auscultation

   1. Perform complete assessment, including Leopold's maneuvers to determine fetal position and palpating the fundus to determine appropriate site for auscultation

   2. Apply fetoscope or Doppler device to the appropriate site

   3. Palpate uterine contractions for frequency, duration, and intensity; confirm uterine rest between contractions; determine if abnormal findings are present

   4. Identify and determine the baseline fetal heart rate and rhythm

   5. Identify the presence of fetal heart rate changes with or between uterine contractions

   6. Determine if findings are reassuring or nonreasurring and implement appropriate nursing interventions, including additional fetal monitoring methods

   7. Identify the clinical situations, based on fetal heart monitoring findings, in which immediate notification of the primary health care provider is appropriate

   8. Communicate the findings from auscultation, interpretation of findings, and resulting nurse intervention(s) in written and verbal form in an appropriate and timely manner

   9. Document appropriate entries on the written or computerized patient record

  10. Demonstrate appropriate maintenance of auscultation equipment

E. Demonstrate use of electronic fetal monitor

   1. Perform complete assessment, including Leopold's maneuvers, palpate the fundus, and auscultate the fetal heart rate before application of thetransducers

   2. Apply external transducers, and adjust the electronic fetal monitor accordingly

3. Prepare the patient, set up the equipment, and complete connections for the fetal electrode with and without intrauterine pressure catheter
4. Calibrate the monitor for the use of the intrauterine pressure catheter
5. Identify technically inadequate tracings, and take appropriate corrective action
6. Obtain and maintain an adequate tracing of the fetal heart and uterine contractions
7. Interpret uterine contraction frequency, duration, intensity, and baseline resting tone as appropriate, based on monitoring method, and determine if abnormal findings are present
8. Identify baseline fetal heart rate and rhythm, variability, and the presence of periodic and nonperiodic changes
9. Determine if findings are reassuring or nonreassuring and implement appropriate nursing interventions
10. Identify the clinical situations, based on fetal heart monitoring findings, in which immediate notification of the primary health care provider is appropriate
11. Communicate the content of electronic fetal monitoring data, interpretation of data, and resulting nursing intervention(s) in written and verbal form in an appropriate and timely manner
12. Document appropriate entries in the written or computerized patient record and on the electronic fetal monitoring tracing or storage disk
13. Demonstrate appropriate maintenance of electronic fetal monitoring equipment
14. Demonstrate appropriate storage and retrieval of fetal heart monitoring data

Educational Guidelines

The content of educational programs specific to intrapartum fetal heart monitoring should include didactic instruction to meet nursing practice competencies, followed by a period of supervised clinical experience before independent nursing practice. The format for presenting didactic instruction may vary, depending on content objectives. A minimum of 8 hours is recommended to cover the core instructional content.

The period of supervised clinical experience required to achieve competency may vary with the individual. As with the core content, ongoing instructional programs may be adapted as necessary to accommodate instructors' and individual learners' needs.

Didactic content outline

I. Introduction to fetal heart monitoring
   A. Goals of fetal heart monitoring
      1. Determine fetal heart rate characteristics and uterine activity
      2. Assess fetal well-being
   B. Methods of monitoring
      1. Auscultation and palpation
      2. Electronic fetal monitoring
         (a) Continuous
         (b) Intermittent
      3. Combination of methods
II. Elements of instrumentation and assessment
   A. Uterine activity monitoring
      1. Palpation
         (a) Principles
         (b) Techniques
         (c) Sources of error and limitations
         (d) Benefits and risks
      2. External electronic: tocodynamometer
         (a) Principles
         (b) Application and care during use
         (c) Sources of error and limitations
         (d) Benefits and risks
      3. Internal electronic: intrauterine pressure catheter
         (a) Types and principles
            (1) Fluid-filled catheters
            (2) Transducer-tipped catheters
         (b) Application and care during use
         (c) Calibration
         (d) Sources of error
         (e) Benefits and risks
   B. Fetal heart rate
      1. External: auscultation
         (a) Types and principles
            (1) Doppler
            (2) Fetoscope
         (b) Techniques

          (c) Sources of error and limitations
          (d) Benefits and risks
      2. External electronic: ultrasound transducer
          (a) Principles of Doppler/ultrasound
          (b) Application and care during use
          (c) Sources of error and limitations
          (d) Benefits and risks
      3. Internal electronic: fetal electrode
          (a) Principles of cardiotachometry
          (b) Application and care during use
          (c) Sources of error and limitations
          (d) Benefits and risks
  C. Equipment maintenance
III. Fetal oxygenation
  A. Physiology of fetal oxygenation
      1. Uteroplacental circulation
      2. Exchange mechanisms
      3. Effects of uterine contractions
      4. Acid-base homeostasis
  B. Pathophysiology of fetal oxygenation
      1. Maternal
          (a) Impaired circulation
          (b) Impaired oxygen exchange
      2. Uterine contraction
          (a) Endogenous causes
          (b) Exogenous causes
      3. Placental
          (a) Impaired circulation
          (b) Impaired oxygen exchange
      4. Umbilical cord
          (a) Compression
          (b) Occlusion
          (c) Compromised perfusion
      5. Fetal
          (a) Impaired circulation
          (b) Impaired oxygen exchange
IV. Interpretation of fetal heart monitoring data
  A. Uterine activity
      1. Resting tone
      2. Contraction frequency

3. Contraction duration
4. Contraction intensity
B. Baseline fetal heart rate and rhythm
    1. Rate and rhythm
        (a) Mechanism (intrinsic and extrinsic control)
            (1) Nervous system control
            (2) Myocardial control
            (3) Endocrine control
            (4) Gestational age influence
        (b) Interpretation
            (1) Normal
            (2) Abnormal
                (a) Tachycardia
                (b) Bradycardia
                (c) Dysrhythmia/Arrhythmia
                (d) Sinusoidal and pseudosinusoidal*
    2. Variability* short- and long-term
        (a) Mechanism
        (b) Interpretation
            (1) Reassuring
            (2) Nonreassuring
C. Periodic fetal heart rate changes*
    1. Accelerations
        (a) Characteristics
        (b) Mechanisms
        (c) Significance
    2. Early decelerations
        (a) Characteristics
        (b) Mechanisms
        (c) Significance
    3. Late decelerations
        (a) Characteristics
        (b) Mechanisms
        (c) Significance
    4. Variable decelerations
        (a) Characteristics
        (b) Mechanisms
        (c) Significance

* Electronic fetal monitoring only.

　　　　5. Prolonged decelerations
　　　　　　(a) Characteristics
　　　　　　(b) Mechanisms
　　　　　　(c) Significance
　　D. Nonperiodic fetal heart rate changes*
　　　　1. Accelerations
　　　　　　(a) Characteristics
　　　　　　(b) Mechanisms
　　　　　　(c) Significance
　　　　2. Variable decelerations
　　　　　　(a) Characteristics
　　　　　　(b) Mechanisms
　　　　　　(c) Significance
　　　　3. Prolonged decelerations
　　　　　　(a) Characteristics
　　　　　　(b) Mechanisms
　　　　　　(c) Significance
　　E. Auscultated fetal heart changes
　　　　1. Numerical rate
　　　　2. Rhythm
　　　　3. Gradual increase or decrease
　　　　4. Abrupt increase or decrease
　V. Nursing process
　　A. Assessment
　　　　1. Review of prenatal history
　　　　2. Clinical status of the mother and fetus
　　　　3. Fetal heart rate characteristics and interpretation
　　　　4. Uterine contraction characteristics and interpretation
　　　　5. Documentation
　　B. Diagnosis
　　　　1. Reassuring
　　　　2. Nonreassuring
　　C. Planning and intervention
　　　　1. Independent nursing actions
　　　　2. Fetal heart monitoring findings necessitating immediate
　　　　　 notification of primary health-care provider

---

* Electronic fetal monitoring only.

      3. Documentation
      4. Nursing accountability
        (a) Policies, procedures, and protocols
        (b) Standards of practice
        (c) Legal and ethical issues
        (d) Lines of authority and responsibility (chain of command)
   D. Evaluation
      1. Response to intervention
      2. Documentation
      3. Continuing plan of nursing care based on response to intervention

Clinical learning experiences and evaluation

The suggested clinical learning experiences and evaluation exercises (pp. 235-236 under "Antepartum Fetal Surveillance") are also appropriate techniques to achieve competency in intrapartum fetal heart monitoring.

Competency Validation

The suggested competency validation exercises (p. 236 under "Antepartum Fetal Surveillance") are also appropriate techniques to validate competency in intrapartum fetal heart monitoring.

Summary

This document provides guidelines for educational preparation to achieve competency in fetal heart monitoring. Nurses should participate annually in reviews and clinical update sessions to maintain competency in fetal heart monitoring. Participation in the clinical learning experiences (pp. 235-236) is encouraged. Maintaining the quality of individual practice in accordance with current guidelines and standards is an inherent responsibility of the professional nurse.

Resources

To obtain information on NAACOG resources regarding fetal heart monitoring, call the NAACOG Fulfillment Department at 1-800-673-8499, extension 2464, or from Canada, 1-800-245-0231, extension 2464.

To obtain information on current ACOG resources addressing fetal monitoring and surveillance, contact the ACOG Resource Center at 1-800-673-8499, extension 2518, or from Canada, 1-800-245-0231, extension 2518.

As a benefit of NAACOG membership, you may request a search of the literature on any topic, including fetal surveillance and fetal heart monitoring. Contact the ACOG Resource Center at 1-800-673-8499, extension 2518, or from Canada, 1-800-245-0231, extension 2518.

This publication was developed by a NAACOG ad hoc committee as a resource to OGN nursing. Guidelines are reviewed every 5 years and revised if necessary. These guidelines do not define a standard of care, and they are not intended to dictate exclusive courses of practice. These guidelines present general, recognized recommendations that are intended to provide a foundation and direction for specialty nursing practice. Variations and innovations that demonstrably improve the quality of patient care are to be encouraged rather than restricted. Guidelines do not replace the NAACOG Standards, but rather expand on the principles suggested therein.

Task Force Members
Chair
Bonnie Flood Chez, RNC, MSN

Members
Catherine Driscoll, RN, BSN
Judy Schmidt, RNC, EdD

Nursing Practice Competencies and Educational Guidelines: Antepartum Fetal Surveillance and Intrapartum Fetal Heart Monitoring has been reviewed by NAACOG members who were designated as nurse consultants. They were selected because of their expertise in fetal surveillance and fetal monitoring. In addition, these guidelines have been reviewed and approved by the NAACOG Committee on Practice. We are indebted to all who shared their time and expertise in the development of this resource.

Glossary of Terms and Abbreviations

abruptio placentae premature separation of the placenta before delivery of the fetus

acceleration transient increase in the fetal heart rate

acidemia increased concentration of hydrogen ions in the blood

acidosis a pathological condition marked by an increased concentration of hydrogen ions in tissue

AFI amniotic fluid index

amniocentesis procedure in which amniotic fluid is removed from the uterine cavity by insertion of a needle through the abdominal and uterine walls into the amniotic sac

amnioinfusion replacement of amniotic fluid with normal saline through an intrauterine pressure catheter

amnion inner of the two fetal membranes forming the sac that encloses the fetus within the uterus

amniotomy artificial rupture of the amniotic sac

anencephaly absence of the cerebrum, cerebellum, and flat bones of the skull

angiography x-ray examination of blood vessels made radiopaque by the injection of a radiopaque substance

antepartum occurring before birth

Apgar score quantitative estimate of the condition of an infant at 1 and 5 minutes after birth, derived by assigning points to the quality of heart rate, respiratory effort, color, muscle tone, and response to stimulation; expressed as the sum of these points with the maximum, or best, score being 10

AROM artificial rupture of membranes

artifact irregularities on a fetal monitor tracing caused by electrical interference or poor reception of the fetal heart rate signal; may appear as scattered dots or lines

ASAP as soon as possible

asphyxia   condition in which there is hypoxia and metabolic acidosis

AST   acoustic stimulation test

atelectasis   collapse of the alveoli, or air sacs, of the lungs

baroceptor   a pressure receptor; a nerve ending located in the walls of the carotid sinus and the aortic arch that is sensitive to stretching induced by changes in blood pressure

baseline FHR   range of FHR present between periodic changes over a 10-minute period

bilirubin   pigment produced by the breakdown of hemoglobin in cell elements and in red blood cells

biparietal diameter   distance from one parietal eminence to another; can be measured by ultrasound to determine gestational age

BP   blood pressure

BPP   biophysical profile

bpm   beats per minute

bradycardia   baseline FHR below 120 bpm for 10 minutes

CC   cord compression

C/C/+1   used to indicate results of vaginal exam (e.g., cervix completely effaced/completely dilated/+1 station)

cephalopelvic disproportion (CPD)   disparity between the size of the fetal head and the maternal pelvis, preventing vaginal delivery

chain-of-command   a reporting mechanism to resolve conflicts

chemoceptor   sensory end organ capable of reacting to a chemical stimulus

chorion   outer of the two membranes forming the sac that encloses the fetus within the uterus

chromosome   a dark stained body within the cell nucleus that carries hereditary factors (genes); there are 46 chromosomes in each cell except in the mature ovum and sperm, where that number is halved

circumvallate placenta   placenta in which an overgrowth of the decidua separates the placental margin from the chorionic plate, producing a thick, white ring around the circumference of the placenta and a reduction in distribution of fetal blood vessels to the placental periphery

cm   centimeter

CNS   central nervous system

CST   contraction stress test

d/c or D/C   discontinue(d)

deceleration   a drop in the FHR; usually occurs in response to a uterine contraction

DIL   cervical dilatation

Doppler ultrasound   type of ultrasound that is reflected from moving interfaces such as closure of fetal heart valves; Doppler ultrasound is used in electronic fetal heart rate monitors

DR   delivery room

ECG   electrocardiogram

EFF   effacement of the cervix

effleurage   gentle stroking of the abdomen; used during labor in the Lamaze method of prepared childbirth

EFM   electronic fetal monitor(ing)

epidural   area situated on or over the dura mater; regional anesthetic is often injected into the peridural (epidural) space of the spinal cord

FBM   fetal breathing movements

FECG   fetal electrocardiogram

FHR   fetal heart rate

FHT   fetal heart tones

FM   fetal movement

FMP   fetal movement profile

frequency (of contractions)   time from the onset of one contraction to the onset of the next or peak of one UC to the peak of the next

FT   fetal tone

gestation   pregnancy; the period of intrauterine fetal development from conception to birth

gestational age   age of a conceptus computed from the first day of the last menstrual period to any point in time thereafter

gtt   drops

HC   head compression

HR   heart rate

hydramnios   excessive volume of amniotic fluid, usually greater than 1.2 L; it is frequently seen in diabetic pregnancies and in fetuses with open neural tube defects

hydrocephaly   increased accumulation of cerebrospinal fluid within the ventricles of the brain; may result from congenital anomalies, infection, injury, or brain tumor; the head is usually large and globular with a disproportionately small face; the increased head diameter is possible in the fetus and infant because the sutures of the skull have not closed

hydrostatic pressure   pressure created in a fluid system

hyperthermia   hyperpyrexia; high fever

hypertonic   solution with a high osmotic pressure

hypertonus   excessive muscular tonus or tension

hypothermia   subnormal temperature of the body

hypotonic   solution with a low osmotic pressure

hypoxemia   decreased oxygen content in the blood

hypoxia   a pathologic condition marked by a decreased level of oxygen in tissue

intervillous space   space between the myometrium and placental villi, which is filled with maternal blood

intrapartum   occurring during labor or delivery

IUP   intrauterine pressure

IUPC   intrauterine pressure catheter

IV   intravenous (parenteral fluids)

L   liter

macrosomia   large body size as seen in some postmature infants and in those born to diabetic mothers

MECG   maternal electrocardiogram

meconium   pasty greenish mass that collects in the fetal intestine, usually expelled during the first 3 to 4 days after birth; its presence in amniotic fluid is abnormal and is usually considered a sign of fetal distress

meningomyelocele   protrusion of a portion of the spinal cord and membranes through a defect in the vertebral column

MHR   maternal heart rate

min   minutes

mm Hg   millimeters of mercury (unit of measure of pressure)

morbidity   state of being diseased or sick; the number of sick persons or cases of disease in relationship to a specific population

mortality   the death rate; the ratio of number of deaths to a given population

mU   milliunits (unit of oxytocin dosage)

nadir   the lowest point of a curve or FHR deceleration

NST   nonstress test

nuchal   neck (as in umbilical cord around the fetal neck)

OCT   oxytocin challenge test

osmolality   quantity of a solute existing in solution as molecules or ions or both; the concentration of a solution

osmotic pressure   pressure developed when two solutions of different concentrations of the same solute are separated by a membrane permeable to the solvent only

PAC   premature atrial contraction

PCB   paracervical block anesthesia

PE   pelvic exam

periodic changes   change in the FHR from the baseline that occurs intermittently

piezoelectric   a substance that has the ability to convert energy from one form into another, such as mechanical pressure into electrical energy and vice versa, as with the ultrasound transducer

PIH   pregnancy-induced hypertension

Pit   Pitocin (oxytocin)

placenta previa   placenta covering the internal cervical os

polyhydramnios   *see* **hydramnios**

prn   as necessary

PROM   premature rupture of membranes

PVC   premature ventricular contraction

q   every

resting tone   intrauterine pressure between contractions (tonus)

R/O   rule out, consider as a possibility

ROM   rupture of membranes

sec   seconds

sinusoidal HR pattern   baseline FHR that has a predominance of long-term variability with a characteristic sine wave pattern

spina bifida   congenital defect in the closure of the vertebral canal with a herniated protrusion of the meninges of the cord

spinal anesthesia   anesthesia produced by the injection of an anesthetic into the spinal subarachnoid space

SROM   spontaneous rupture of membranes

STA   station

supine hypotension   weight and pressure of uterus on the ascending vena cava when the patient is in a supine position decreases venous return, cardiac output, and blood pressure

surfactant   phospholipid that normally lines the alveolar sacs after 34 weeks gestation. Its presence prevents collapse (atelectasis) of the alveoli by permitting a small amount of air to remain in the alveoli on exhalation. The L/S ratio as measured in amniotic fluid tests for the presence of surfactant. Neonates born without surfactant develop respiratory distress syndrome (RDS)

SVT   supraventricular tachycardia

tachycardia   baseline FHR above 160 bpm for 10 minutes

tachysystole   excessive uterine contraction frequency

tetany   state of increased neuromuscular irritability or spasm

toco   tocotransducer or tocodynamometer, external device used to record uterine activity

tocodynamometer   pressure-sensing instrument for measuring the duration and frequency of uterine contractions

tocolytics   drugs used to inhibit uterine contractions and stop labor

tocotransducer   *see* **tocodynamometer**

tonus   intrauterine pressure between contractions (resting tone)

transducer   device that converts energy from one form to another; sound or pressure can be converted into an electrical impulse and vice versa

UA   uterine activity

UC   uterine contraction

ultrasound transducer   instrument that uses high-frequency sound (ultrasound) to detect moving interfaces, such as the closure of fetal heart valves, to monitor the fetal heart rate

UPI   uteroplacental insufficiency

US   ultrasound

variability   fluctuations in the baseline FHR

VAS   vibroacoustic stimulation

VBAC   vaginal birth after cesarean

VE   vaginal exam

Bibliography

Afriat CI: Historical perspective on electronic fetal monitoring: A decade of growth, a decade of conflict, *J Perinat Neonatal Nurs* 1(1):1-4, 1987.

Afriat CI: *Electronic fetal monitoring,* Rockville, Md, 1989, Aspen Publishers.

American Academy of Pediatrics and American College of Obstetricians and Gynecologists: *Guidelines for perinatal care,* Washington, DC, 1992, The Academy and The College.

American College of Obstetricians and Gynecologists: *Assessment of fetal and newborn acid-base status,* Technical Bulletin No 127, Washington, DC, April 1989, The College.

American College of Obstetricians and Gynecologists: *Intrapartum fetal heart rate monitoring,* ACOG Technical Bulletin No 132, Washington, DC, September 1989, The College.

American College of Obstetricians and Gynecologists: *Prostaglandin E_2 gel for cervical ripening,* ACOG Committee Opinion 123, Washington, DC, 1993, The College.

American College of Obstetricians and Gynecologists: *Antepartum fetal surveillance,* Technical Bulletin, 1994, The College.

Association of Women's Health, Obstetric, and Neonatal Nurses: *Cervical ripening and induction and augmentation of labor,* Practice resource, Washington, DC, 1993, The Association.

Association of Women's Health, Obstetric and Neonatal Nurses: *Fetal heart monitoring principles and practice,* Washington, DC, 1993, The Association.

Auyeung RM, Goldkrand JW: Vibroacoustic stimulation and nursing intervention in the nonstress test, *JOGNN* 20(3):232-238, 1991.

Bald R et al: Antepartum fetal blood sampling with cordocentesis: Comparison with chorionic villus sampling and amniocentesis in diagnosing karyotype anomalies, *J Reprod Med* 36(9)655-658, 1991.

Benn PA et al: Prenatal diagnosis of diverse chromosome abnormalities in a population of patients identified by triple-marker testing as screen positive for Down Syndrome, *Am J Obstet Gynecol* 173(2):496-501, 1995.

Berkus M et al: Meconium-stained amniotic fluid: Increased risk for adverse neonatal outcome, *Obstet Gynecol* 84(1):115-120, 1994.

Besinger RE, Johnson TRB: Doppler recordings of fetal movement: Clinical correlation with real-time ultrasound, *Obstet Gynecol* 74:277-280, 1989.

Bevis DCA: The antenatal prediction of haemolytic disease of the newborn, *Lancet* I:395-398, Feb 1952.

Cabaniss ML: *Fetal monitoring interpretation,* Philadelphia, 1993, JB Lippincott.

Capeless EL, Mann LI: Use of breast stimulation for antepartum stress testing, *Obstet Gynecol* 64(5):641-645, 1984.

Centers for Disease Control and Prevention: Mortality patterns: United States and infant mortality: United States: 1992, *JAMA* 273(2)100-101, 1995.

Clark S, Sabey P, Jolley K: Nonstress testing with acoustic stimulation and amniotic volume assessment: 5973 tests without unexpected fetal death, *Am J Obstet Gynecol* 160:694, 1989.

Clark SL: Do we still need fetal scalp blood sampling? *Contemp Ob/Gyn* 33(3):75-86, 1989.

Clark SL: How a modified NST improves fetal surveillance, *Contemp Ob/Gyn* 35(5):45-48, 1990.

Clark SL, Cotton DB, Editors: *Critical care obstetrics,* Boston, 1991, Blackwell Scientific Publications.

Clements JA, Platzker ACG, Tierney DF: Assessment of the risk of the respiratory distress syndrome by a rapid test for surfactant in amniotic fluid, *N Engl J Med* 286:1077, 1972.

Chez BF: *EFM terminology: communicating if you are reassured or not,* Third Annual National Conference of Electronic Fetal Monitoring: The Science, the Art, the Future, October 1992.

Chez BF: Electronic fetal monitoring competency—To validate or not to validate: The opinion of experts, *J Perinat Neonatal Nurs* 8(3):9-12, 1994.

Childress CH, Katz VL: Nifedipine and its indications in obstetrics and gynecology, *Obstet Gynecol* 83(4):616-624, 1994.

Davis LK: Nursing care protocols and procedures. In Mandeville LK, Troiano NH, eds: *High-risk intrapartum nursing,* Philadelphia, 1992, JB Lippincott.

Dicker D et al: Effect of intracranial pressure changes on the fetal heart rate: Study of a hydrocephalic fetus, *Israel J Med Sci* 19:364, 1983.

Didolkar S, Mutch M: Major/multiple congenital anomalies and intrapartum fetal heart rate pattern, *South Dakota J Med* 39:5, 1979.

Freeman RK, Garite TJ, Nageotte MP: *Fetal heart rate monitoring,* Baltimore, 1991, Williams & Wilkins.

Gaffney SE, Salinger L, Vintzileos AM: The biophysical profile for fetal surveillance, *MCN* 15(6):356-360, 1990.

Gegor CL, Paine LL: Antepartum fetal testing techniques: An update for today's perinatal nurse, *J Perinat Neonatal Nurs* 5(4):1-15, 1992.

Gilstrap LC et al: Diagnosis of birth asphyxia on the basis of fetal pH, Apgar score, and newborn cerebral dysfunction, *Am J Obstet Gynecol* 161:825, 1989.

Gluck L et al: Diagnosis of respiratory distress syndrome by amniocentesis, *Am J Obstet Gynecol* 109(3):441, 1971.

Goff v. Doctors Hospital, 166 Cal App. 314,333 P.2d, 29, 1958.

Hankins GDV: Apgar scores: Are they enough? *Contemp Ob/Gyn:Ob-Gyn Law Special Issue* 36:13-25, 1991.

Haverkamp AD et al: The evaluation of continuous fetal heart rate monitoring in high risk pregnancy, *Am J Obstet Gynecol* 123:310, 1976.

Haverkamp AD et al: A controlled trial of the differential effects of intrapartum fetal monitoring, *Am J Obstet Gynecol* 134(4):399-412, 1979.

Heppart MCS, Garite TJ: Acute obstetrics: A practical guide, St. Louis, 1992, Mosby.

Hon Edward H: *An introduction to fetal heart rate monitoring,* Wallingford, Conn, 1975 (Distributed by Corometrics).

Huddleston JF: Contraction stress test by intermittent nipple stimulation, *Obstet Gynecol* 63(5):669-673, 1984.

Iams JD, Johnson FF, Parker M: A prospective evaluation of the signs and symptoms of preterm labor, *Obstet Gynecol* 84(2):227-230, 1994.

Kirshon B et al: Influence of short-term indomethacin therapy on fetal urine output, *Obstet Gynecol* 72:51, 1988.

Leveno KJ et al: A prospective comparison of selective and universal electronic fetal monitoring in 34,995 pregnancies, *N Engl J Med* 315:615, 1986.

Luttkus et al: Continuous monitoring of fetal oxygen saturation by pulse oximetry, *Obstet Gynecol* 85(2):183-186, 1995.

Manning FA et al: Fetal biophysical profile scoring: Selective use of the nonstress test, *Am J Obstet Gynecol* 156(3):709-712, 1987.

Manning FA et al: Fetal assessment based on fetal biophysical profile scoring. IV. An analysis of perinatal morbidity and mortality, *Am J Obstet Gynecol* 162:703, 1990.

Marci CJ et al: Prophylactic amnioinfusion improves outcome of pregnancy complicated by thick meconium and oligohydramnios, *Am J Obstet Gynecol* 167, 117-121, 1992.

McNamara H, Johnson N, Lilford R: The effect on fetal arteriolar oxygen saturation resulting from giving oxygen to the mother measured by pulse oximetry, *Br J Obstet Gynaecol,* 100:446-449, 1993.

McRae MJ: Litigation, electronic fetal monitoring and the obstetric nurse, *JOGNN* 22(5):410-419, 1993.

Melendez TD, Rayburn WF, Smith CV: Characterization of fetal body movement recorded by the Hewlett-Packard M-1350-A fetal monitor, *Am J Obstet Gynecol* 166:700-702, 1992.

Menticoglou S et al: Severe fetal brain injury without intrapartum asphyxia or trauma, *Obstet Gynecol* 74:457, 1989.

Miller LA: Electronic fetal monitoring competency—To validate or not to validate: The opinions of experts, *J Perinat Neonatal Nurs* 8(3):12-15, 1994.

Miyasaki FS, Nevarez F: Saline amnioinfusion for relief of repetitive variable decelerations: A prospective randomized study, *Am J Obstet Gynecol* 153(3):301-306, 1985.

Miyasaki FS, Taylor NA: Saline amnioinfusion for relief of variable or prolonged decelerations, *Am J Obstet Gynecol* 146(6):670-678, 1983.

Mooney RA et al: Effectiveness of combining maternal serum alpha-feto-protein and hCG in a second-trimester screening program for Down syndrome, *Obstet Gynecol* 83(6):298, 1994.

Moore TR: Superiority of the four-quadrant sum over the single-deepest-pocket technique in ultrasonographic identification of abnormal amniotic fluid volumes, *Am J Obstet Gynecol* 163:762, 1990.

Murray M: *Antepartal and intrapartal fetal monitoring,* Washington, DC, 1988, Nurses Association of the American College of Obstetricians and Gynecologists (NAACOG).

Niebyl JR, Witter FR: Neonatal outcome after indomethacin treatment for preterm labor, *Am J Obstet Gynecol* 155:747-9, 1986.

Niswander KR: EFM and brain damage in term and post-term infants, *Contemp Ob/Gyn: Ob/Gyn Law Special Issue* 36:39-50, 1991.

Nocon JJ: Risk management and neurologically impaired infants, *Contemp Ob/Gyn* 36 (Special Issue) 61-68, Feb 15, 1991.

Nurses Association of the American College of Obstetricians and Gynecologists: *Fetal heart rate auscultation,* OGN nursing practice resource, Washington, DC, March 1990, NAACOG: The Organization for Obstetric, Gynecologic and Neonatal Nurses.

Nurses Association of the American College of Obstetricians and Gynecologists: Nursing practice competencies and educational guidelines: Antepartum fetal surveillance and intrapartum fetal heart rate monitoring, Washington, DC, 1991, The Association.

Nurses Association of the American College of Obstetricians and Gynecologists: *Standards for obstetric, gynecologic, and neonatal nursing,* ed 4, Washington, DC, 1991, The Association.

Nurses Association of the American College of Obstetricians and Gynecologists: Statement: nursing responsibilities in implementing intrapartum fetal heart rate monitoring, Washington, DC, 1992, The Association.

Ombelet W, VanDerMerwe J: Sinusoidal fetal heart rate pattern associated with congenital hydrocephalus, *S Afr Med J* 67:423, 1985.

Orimi v. Mission Viejo Hospital, Orange County Superior Court, *Professional Liability Newsletter,* March 1985.

Page FO et al: Correlation of neonatal acid-base status with Apgar scores and fetal heart rate tracings, *Am J Obstet Gynecol* 154(6):1306-1310, 1986.

Parer JT: *Handbook of fetal heart rate monitoring,* Philadelphia, 1983, WB Saunders.

Parer JT: *Physiology of FHR patterns,* Course syllabus for antepartum and intrapartum management, San Francisco, 1991, 183-204.

Parer JT: *Continuous electronic fetal monitoring in labor,* Course syllabus for a comprehensive fetal heart rate monitoring training program, San Francisco, 1993.

Platt LD: Predicting fetal health with the biophysical profile, *Contemp Ob/Gyn* 33(2):105-119, 1989.

Rabello YA, Lapidus MR: *Fundamentals of electronic fetal monitoring,* Wallingford, Conn, 1991, Corometric Medical Systems.

Rubsamen DS: The obstetrician's professional liability: Awareness and prevention, Professional Liability Newsletter, Inc, 1993, Orange County Superior Court, No 30-29-74.

Rutherford SE et al: The four-quadrant assessment of amniotic fluid volume: An adjunct to antepartum fetal heart rate testing, *Obstet Gynecol* 70:353, 1987.

Saling E, Schneider D: Biochemical supervision of the foetus during labour, *J Obstet Gynecol Br Commonwealth* 74:749, 1967.

Schifrin BS, Weissman BA, Wiley J: Electronic fetal monitoring and obstetrical malpractice, *Law, Medicine and Health Care* 13(3), June 1985.

Schmidt J: *Cervical ripening and induction and augmentation of labor,* AWHONN Practice Resource, Washington, DC, 1993.

Shy KK, Larson EB, Luthy DA: Evaluating a new technology: The effectiveness of electronic fetal heart rate monitoring, *Annu Rev Public Health* 8:165-190, 1987.

Sleutel MR: An overview of vibrocoustic stimulation, *JOGNN* 18(6):447-452, Nov/Dec 1989.

Smith CV et al: Fetal acoustic stimulation testing: A randomized clinical comparison with the nonstress test, *Am J Obstet Gynecol* 155(1):131-134, 1986.

Stanco LM et al: Does Doppler-detected fetal movement decrease the incidence of nonreactive nonstress tests? *Obstet Gynecol* 82(6):999-103, 1993.

Stringer M et al: Maternal-fetal physical assessment in the home setting: Role of the advanced practice nurse, *JOGNN* 23(8):720-725, 1994.

Thorp JA et al: Routine umbilical cord blood gas determinations? *Am J Obstet Gynecol* 161:600, 1989.

Trofatter KF: Cervical ripening, *Clin Obstet Gynecol* 35:476, 1992.

Umstad MP, Permzel M, Pepperell RJ: Litigation and the intrapartum cardiotocograph, *Br J Obstet Gynaecol* 102:89-91, 1995.

VanderMoer P, Gerretsen G, Visser G: Fixed fetal heart rate pattern after intrauterine accidental decerebration, *Obstet Gynecol* 65:125, 1985.

Vintzileos AM et al: A randomized trial of intrapartum electronic fetal heart rate monitoring versus intermittent auscultation, *Obstet Gynecol* 81(6):899-907, 1993.

Wallerstedt C et al: Amnioinfusion: An update, *JOGNN* 23(7):573-577, 1994.

Yoon BH et al: Relationship between the fetal biophysical profile score, umbilical artery Doppler velocimetry and fetal blood acid-base status determined by cordocentesis, *Am J Obstet Gynecol* 169(6), 1586-94, 1993.

Index